G000253443

The Importa
Dads and Grandmas to the
Breastfeeding Mother

UK Version

Wendy Jones, PhD, MRPharmS

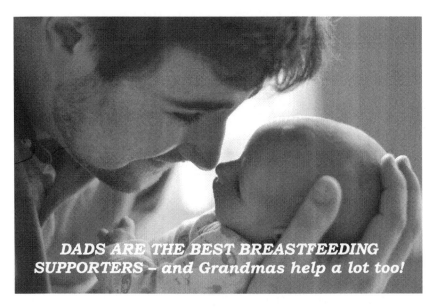

DADS ARE THE BEST BREASTFEEDING SUPPORTERS – and Grandmas help a lot too!

Praeclarus Press, LLC

www.PraeclarusPress.com

Praeclarus Press, LLC

2504 Sweetgum Lane

Amarillo, Texas 79124 USA

806-367-9950

www.PraeclarusPress.com

DISCLAIMER

The information contained in this publication is advisory only and is not
intended to replace sound clinical judgment or individualized patient care.
The author disclaims all warranties, whether expressed or implied, including
any warranty as the quality, accuracy, safety, or suitability of this information
for any particular purpose.

ISBN: 978-1-939807-92-2

Cover Design and Production: Ken Tackett

Developmental Editing: Kathleen Kendall-Tackett

Copy Editing: Chris Tackett

Layout & Design: Nelly Murariu

This book is dedicated to three very important people in my life: my daughter, my son-in-law, and my grandson, who became a family in June, 2013. They taught me so much more about breastfeeding than all the theory I had learned in the past 25 years, and from a very different perspective to that of being a mum myself.

Sadly, this wonderful and precious family was to have to bear the tragic loss of Christian, who died on October 1st 2013, following a very brief, but courageously fought battle against metastatic colorectal cancer. During the 42 days that Christian was in hospital, Kerensa stayed by his side whilst continuing to breastfeed Stirling. No one ever asked her to take the baby away. In fact, he was petted and adored by all the staff. Despite everything that happened in these traumatic weeks, Kerensa's milk supply remained high due, we believe, to the love that they shared as a couple.

Even having to return to full-time work with a 4-month-old baby in daycare did not stop her from exclusively breast-feeding Stirling for 6 months. I am so proud of these three very special people. This book has been written as a tribute to them. Their story has been included to illustrate the breastfeeding journey. I have shared some of the precious photographs that we took during the special time they had together.

Jon Christian Klottrup was a wonderful father who will never be forgotten. This book is a celebration of his life as a father.

If fatherhood doesn't mean feeding, what does it mean? Everything else!

Diane Wiessinger, MS, IBCLC

Common sense is not so common.

Voltaire, Dictionnaire Philosophique, 1764

When asked how he felt about watching his wife breastfeed, my son-in-law (an IT expert) said:

It's like finding out that my favourite software package has free, bonus features.

Acknowledgements

Thank you to Juliet Klottrup for some fabulous illustrations, to Jenny Richardson and Carolyn Wetscott for giving me permission to use your drawings and photographs again, and to Charlotte Raw and Laura Legg for your constructive comments. Thank you also, Gill and Rob Klottrup, for letting me tell the story of your wonderful son, whom we all miss every day.

I can't pass up this opportunity to express my eternal gratitude to my husband of 40 years for not only putting up with my passion, but encouraging me. Last, but very much not least, my three wonderful daughters, Kerensa, Bethany, and Tara, for teachingme so much every day since they were born.

CONTENTS

WHEN A BREASTFEEDING MOTHER MAY NEED TO TAKE MEDICINE

Background

I have spent the last 25 years teaching and supporting breastfeeding, culminating in the publication of a book called Breastfeeding and Medication in 2013. I am committed to providing evidence-based information and helping women to make the choices that are right for them. But now I am a Grandmother. I remember that I was scared by the prospect of supporting my eldest daughter as she became a mother. How could I help her? How could I help my son-in-law? I was there to help her get breastfeeding off to a good start, I hoped!

My daughter's birth took place in a hospital in the USA, where she was living at the time. I hope to use this opportunity to compare and contrast practices in the two countries so we can adopt the best practices of both.

I am hoping to provide information for other grandmothers, and also fathers on how to support the new mother in breastfeeding, and to share some of our experiences and what we learned along the way as we went through this exciting journey.

I guess all of my daughters have an unusual perspective on breastfeeding because they have grown up with hearing me talk about it—as have all my dear son-in-laws. Breastfeeding is a normal topic of conversation in our home. Having heard of all the differences between artificial formula milk and breastmilk, there was never a discussion about doing anything other than breastfeed this precious little bundle we were waiting to greet. By reading this book, I hope that you will understand more about how breastfeeding works from evidence-based studies, and how to encourage the new mother in your life to initiate and continue as long as she and your lovely new baby wish. I hope that I can write this book in a style that meets your needs, as well as those of the woman at the centre of your life.

I am not expecting this to be a book you read from cover-to-cover. Think of it as a toolbox with information on how to fix problems if they occur (and not everyone has problems). Maybe it will stimululate discussion on how you all feel about breastfeeding. Maybe it will be a vehicle to decide what each of you will do when the new baby is born. This may be a first baby, or may be a new baby after a struggle to breastfeed last time. Let me say this now; whatever you did last time, if you stopped sooner than you planned, you did not fail. There is no right or wrong in parenting. We all do the best we have with the knowledge and support we have at that time. Sometimes that knowledge changes and sometimes you learn how to get more support.

Being a parent is not easy and inevitably comes with periods of guilt. I didn't have a natural birth. I didn't enjoy breastfeeding. My baby didn't sleep as well as everyone else's. (I bet that most people lie about how long their baby sleeps.) I didn't get on with baby-led weaning. We didn't have a routine. I had to go back to work/I didn't go back to work. And it goes on. Just enjoy every day with your child and do the best you can. There is no such thing as a perfect parent (or grandparent); good enough will do.

I recently attended a workshop where we were discussing cards with sentences such as "who supports breastfeeding?" "who promotes formula-feeding?" "what do fathers think about breast-feeding?" and "what do grandmothers think about breastfeeding?" written on them. It made me think that there are many variations in the answers. One person commented that grandmothers discourage breastfeeding so that they can feed the baby. Someone else said the same about fathers, but that it was in order to be more involved with the baby. Another person commented that her partner wanted her to breastfeed so he didn't have to get up in the night, but was happy to take over bath-time duties. Whether you chose for your partner to give bottles of expressed milk, to combination feed, or to exclusively breastfeed is your decision.

Breastmilk is infinitely adaptable, making it perfect for your baby in quality and quantity. It varies from day to day, throughout the day, and depending on where in the world the baby is born, and at what gestation. So if a baby is born in the desert, the breastmilk that the mother produces will be waterier. If born in the Arctic, it will contain more fat to keep the baby warm. If the baby is born prematurely, the milk contains more protein to help the baby grow. That is what makes breastmilk so special and a product that formula-milk manufacturers can never reproduce, however big their budgets. It also contains antibodies to any infection that the mother has encountered to protect the baby. Breastfed babies need nothing apart from breastmilk. Even on the hottest summer day, the baby does not need water. Frequent short breastfeeds will meet the baby's thirst.

This book will provide you with information on the impact that may or may not have on breastfeeding, on you, and on your baby. It will give you explanations, but the decisions are yours and not the business of anyone else. The baby is being fed, and that is all that matters. I would be lying if I didn't admit that I hope that it will help you exclusively breastfeed for 6 months, and then continue along with solids as long as you wish. But that is my agenda, not yours!

DADS ARE THE BEST BREASTFEEDING SUPPORTERS - and Grandmas help a lot too!

Support your partner with breastfeeding to ensure your little one has the best start in the game called life.

Breastmilk provides all the goodness that your baby needs for the first 6 months of life. It is also valuable to your baby if he is on solids. Formula milk cannot provide all the special protective factors that nature adds to breastmilk to make it special for your baby. Breastmilk is always available at the right temperature, in the right amount, and the packaging is perfect!

BE A SUPPORTER

Support the BEST team in the world

YOUR TEAM

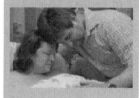

If your partner breastfeeds, your new baby will be at lower risk of:

- ✔ Diarrhoea and other tummy infections
- ✔ Chest Infections
- ✔ Ear Infections
- ✔ Urine infections
- ✔ Asthma
- ✔ Eczema
- ✔ Childhood diabetes
- ✔ Obesity

BUT did you also know?

If your partner breastfeeds, **she** will have a reduced risk of:

- ✔ Breast cancer
- ✔ Ovarian cancer
- ✔ Weak Bones in later life
- ✔ Obesity

AND she will get her figure back faster.

REMIND your partner to call for help from one of the numbers she was given after the baby was born if she:

- Finds breastfeeding painful
- Is concerned that everything isn't going as she expected
- Needs to talk to other mums

So what can YOU do to help?

Some dads feel left out if they can't feed their baby. But breastmilk is protecting your partner and your baby. Isn't that the most important thing?

You can play with your baby, sing (they don't care how much in or out of tune you are or what you sing!), bathe your baby, or just enjoy being together as a family.

You can earn her thanks by bringing her a cup of tea and a snack when she's breastfeeding, of course!

Introduction for Grandma and Dad

How Do You Feel, Grandma?

So Grandma, how does this next stage of growing up feel? Your precious baby daughter or son has announced that she/he is going to be a parent. You are going to be a grandmother! What thoughts spring to your mind? Is it "I'm not old enough to be a grandmother!" or perhaps, "Thank Heavens, I thought this day would never come!" It is inevitably a huge and complex mix of emotions.

For me, it brought back, with amazing clarity, how I felt telling my mum I was pregnant for the first time, almost 35 years ago. Memories of my daughter's birth surfaced for the first time in many years. Isn't it amazing how those early hours with your new baby remain so detailed, but the pain of labour, thankfully, diminishes? The timing of that transition into womanhood was a very special time for me. I can recall those early days (after each birth) in vivid technicolour, and how important the presence and support of my own mum, sadly no longer with us, was to me.

As days, weeks, and months passed during my daughter's pregnancy, I found that our relationship changed subtly. We were no longer were just mum and daughter. We were members of womankind, the keepers of the genetic pool, the givers of life, and the continuation of our family line, even though we were living on opposite sides of the Atlantic Ocean.

I remember so clearly when my new grandchild was 8 days overdue. We are all impatient for the baby to be born, but also slightly apprehensive about the change about to take place in our lives. I felt fiercely protective of my baby; a feeling that I have had all her life (and for her two sisters, I hasten to emphasise). She was entering a new and scary, but also exciting time. I wanted to make it an easy transition. I had to recognise that I had no control. She and her husband had to do this together. I needed to remain in the background, loving them, supporting them, but above all, empowering them to take these new, unfamiliar steps which would make them parents, a step to change their lives forever. It would also change mine and my husband's as we became grandparents.

So Why Do You Need to Read This Book?

If you breastfed your babies, surely the decision is made and you know the practicalities of breastfeeding? Actually, many of the things I was taught as a new mother have changed with the passage of time and better research-based information. I was told to start to feed for 2 minutes, each side gradually increasing to a maximum of 10 minutes for each side, and then to top the baby up with cooled, boiled water. Sometimes I wonder how I managed to breastfeed, and how my baby grew under this regime. Probably because my own mum encouraged me to watch my baby and to respond to her needs, and we threw the rule book out within the first 2 weeks.

Different rules are suggested now, but hopefully, based on evidence. Guidance on when to introduce solid foods has changed dramatically, so you may need to read that section. However, I think just as the recollection of the pain of labour goes, so does the memory of the bad old days. It may be that you never had any problems breastfeeding, but the mum you are supporting is not finding breastfeeding as easy. This book will provide an explanation and some suggestions on how to overcome the difficulties. You may not want to read it from cover to cover, but keep it as a reference tool. Will your knowledge be as welcome if the new mother is your daughter-in-law? Of course it will! Your son has the role of supporting his partner in their new jouney together. Who else will he trust in providing information and support to him in this often very scary, grown-up role?

If you formula milk-fed your babies, why do you need to read this book? Does it feel difficult to even contemplate supporting the mother of your grandchild in her choice of breastfeeding? Are you trying to understand why the new parents have decided to breastfeed? It can be hard as it suggests that they disagree with what you did. Does that imply your decision was wrong? We all make decisions in our children's lives with the best information we had at that time. Thirty years ago, the vast majority of babies were formula-fed from birth, and the upward trend in breastfeeding has been very slow. Thus, we have had a generation of health care professionals who, maybe, didn't breastfeed their own babies, and also have not honed their skills to support breastfeeding. You may have tried, but not managed to breastfeed, or may never have started. That is okay. Don't take the new parents decision as negative to your decision and your childrearing. This is a new baby, about to be born in a different society, to new parents who need every bit of your love, support, and care.

How Do You Feel, Dad?

So, congratulations! You are nearing the end of pregnancy. How are you feeling? A new life about to join your family—a huge responsibility for the next 20 years. I bet you have discussed with other fathers about how they have found fatherhood. I am sure many of those stories were scary. Maybe you have asked your own father what it was like when you were about to be born. You are now the "man of the house," the "guardian of the family," and the "provider and carer." Did you think about this part 9 months ago?

How can you help in this next stage? If your partner has chosen to breastfeed, you might think there's nothing you can do. Let me assure you that there is a lot you can do. Breastfeeding is the best way for a baby to be fed. Everyone has told you that. Research shows that it not only benefits the baby, but also the mother. So why would you not choose this?

Positive attitudes toward breastfeeding from the father are important in a mother's success in initiating and continuing breastfeeding, so you are important! Research suggests that without the support of their partners, women are more likely to choose formula-feeding. It is thought that changing the negative attitudes and perceptions of breastfeeding in partners could be one way to increase breastfeeding rates (Mitchell-Box et al., 2013). Breastfeeding is a team effort. Some people say it takes a whole village to support a breastfeeding mother. It certainly needs a supportive dad.

I don't for one minute expect you to read this whole book! What I do want you to do is remember where you put it, and read the first chapter of why breastfeeding is so special for your partner and your baby. Men are often great problem solvers. When new mothers are desperately tired, we can all lose the plot! We need you to remind us why we chose to breastfed, and why, if things are not going quite according to our plans and dreams, that we may need help. Or we may just need reassurance that babies haven't read their own instruction manual, and don't know the rules to meet our expectations.

In this book, there are lots of problems and how to solve them. I promise that you are not going to encounter all the problems, but I can't write a book just for you. It has to meet everyone's needs. You can find the part of the book that relates to the "problem," and help your partner understand what is going on. You might need help, whether you need to call someone, post on a Facebook group, or email me. Or you just need to relax and know it is okay. Your job may sound simple (my son-in-law thought one of the advantages of breastfeeding was that he didn't need to do anything), but it is actually essential. Your love and support are, as always, integral to the needs of your family. You, our partners, are our supermen. You can spend time with your baby bathing, singing, reading, rocking, or anything else other than feeding (notice I am not saying your role is nappy changing).

This may be your first baby, and you want to do everything perfectly. Or it may be that feeding was difficult, or you didn't try last time, but this time, you and your partner would like to. Even if it is your fifth baby, it will be different for every baby. Each experience is unique. You may feel confident, or you may feel totally out of your depth. I will share stories that make this new journey real from the experience of another man who was once as anxious as you are now.

I am going to refer to the baby as "he" throughout the book, just to make it easier for you to see when I am referring to the mother as "she." Every baby is worth its weight in gold, male or female, and as the mother of 3 daughters and 2 grandsons, I am not in any way biased!

How Does the New Mum Feel?

The new mum in your life may be the one who bought this book and given it to you to read. At every midwife or doctor check-up, it is likely that how she is planning to feed the baby will have been raised. It is a topic of discussion with many pregnant women, and tends to be filled with many horror stories about how difficult it is and how things can go wrong so quickly, leading to pain and destroyed nipples. She may be very anxious, and looking to you both for support. We all want to do the best for our babies, and it is acknowledged, even by mothers who choose to formula-feed, that breastfeeding has advantages.

It is possible that she feels under some pressure to breast-feed because that is what her friends and family have done, or threatened because they haven't done so. If this isn't your first baby—or is maybe the first baby you have had together after the breakup of previous relationships—you need to remember that he is his own little person, and not the same as his brother or sister. If breastfeeding went well last time, that is positive, but it may not be as simple this time. If breastfeeding didn't go so well last time, it is still different and may be easier.

My main message is to discuss what you want from each other, to listen, and respect each other's views, and to love your baby for himself, however he is fed.

WHAT MAKES BREASTMILK SPECIAL?

I could write a whole book just to cover this topic. There is barely a day, even after 30 years of studying breastfeeding, that I don't find something else new which blows my mind.

Protection from Infection

One of the most amazing things about breastmilk, and the inter-action between mother and baby, is the production of antibodies in response to infections in order to protect the baby. If a mother encounters an infection, let us say, as an example, when out shopping, she meets someone with a cold who sneezes viral droplets without covering his/her nose. The mother will have produced antibodies to that infection before the next breastfeed to protect her infant. Even if they both contract the virus, the baby will be significantly less sick than if he had been formula-fed, and hence, not being protected by maternal antibodies. Similarly, if the mother develops a gastrointestinal infection, the baby will be protected in an incredibly short space of time.

Amazingly, saliva changes if the baby meets an infection, inviting mum to make antibodies to it and hence, to protect her child. There are many acknowledged and well-researched reduced risks of infections attributed to exclusive breastfeeding.

- Less risk of gastroenteritis (Howie et al., 1990; Kramer et al., 2003; Quigley et al., 2007; Rebhan et al., 2009; Wilson et al., 1998)

- Fewer middle-ear infections (Aniansson et al., 1994; Duncan et al., 1993)

⊙ Reduction in urinary tract infection (Marild et al., 2004; Pisacane et al., 1992)

⊙ Fewer lower respiratory tract diseases (Bachrach et al., 2003; Ball & Wright, 1999; Howie et al., 1990)

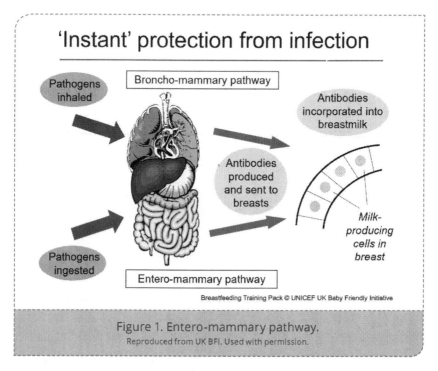

Figure 1. Entero-mammary pathway.
Reproduced from UK BFI. Used with permission.

Many mothers are aware that breastfeeding is healthier for their baby. The Infant Feeding Survey (McAndrew et al., 2012) asked women what had influenced their feeding choice. That breastfeeding was "best for the baby" was cited by 83% of all mothers, with 75% being able to name a benefit without prompting. The second most common reason given was convenience, whilst 17% were also aware of the health benefits for the mother. Most women who were interviewed for the survey were aware that breastfeeding helps to build the baby's immunity, resulting from antibodies passed on from the mother.

Constituents of Breastmilk

Over 200 living constituents of breastmilk have been identified. The content of breastmilk depends on the age of the baby, the time of day, and the interval with the preceding feed. These factors are specific to meet the nutritional needs of the individual infant at that time. Breastmilk is a living fluid which keeps changing from day to day, week to week, and even feed to feed to meet your baby's individual needs. This makes it a magical substance worth its weight in gold.

Constituents of Formula

Formula milk is modified cow's milk (with the exception of some specialised milks necessary for infants with cow's-milk-protein intolerance). Manufactures have an impossible task in developing and marketing their product. They have to produce a standardized, heavily regulated product at an affordable price. Each company seeks to promote their brand by making it appear special and different to their competitors. Brand loyalty is encouraged.

There is no evidence that:

⊙ Any brand of formula milk is superior to any other

⊙ Switching from whey- to casein-dominant milk is necessary

⊙ The introduction to follow-on milks is necessary

⊙ The introduction of specially designed toddler milks is necessary

Manufacturers have great difficulty identifying, let alone reproducing the components of breastmilk. Formula milk is a nutritionally adequate fluid, the content of which is controlled by the internationally agreed regulations. It is used by many families as a part, or total part, of their baby's diet, and there is nothing wrong with that. In the UK, only 2% of babies are exclusively breastfed (no formula milk or other liquids apart from medicines) at 6 months (McAndrew et al., 2012). What I want you to understand is what makes breastmilk special, so you can make an informed decision.

The Health of a Breastfed Baby

The feeding of newborns makes a critical contribution to their short- and long-term health. At no other period in human life is there total dependence on one food to meet all nutritional needs to secure optimal growth and development. Formula milk is a breastmilk substitute. However, we have yet to see much come from it as the normal way to feed babies.

On a population base, infants who are not breastfed show an increased risk of:
Ear Infections (Aniansson et al., 1994; Duncan et al., 1993)
Gastroenteritis (Howie et al., 1990; Kramer et al., 2003; Wilson et al., 1998; Quigley, 2007; Rebhan et al., 2009)
Urinary tract infection (Marild et al., 2004; Pisacane et al., 1992)
Pneumonia (Ip et al., 2007)
Lower Respiratory Tract Infections (Bachrach et al., 2003; Ball et al., 1999; Howie, 1990)
Childhood obesity (Grube et al., 2015; Redsell et al., 2015; Yan et al., 2014)
Type 1 diabetes (Alves et al., 2011)
Type 2 diabetes (Owen et al., 2006)
Leukemia (Amitay et al., 2015; Kwan et al., 2004)
Sudden Infant Death Syndrome (Ip et al., 2007)
Premature infants who are not breastfed are at an increased risk of:
Necrotizing enterocolitis (NEC) (Ip et al., 2007)

Factors in Breastmilk, but Not in Infant Formula

So what is it that is in breastmilk that provides the baby with better health outcomes than those who are formula-fed? How do these factors protect the infant?

Lactoferrin

Lactoferrin is a protein that binds to iron to help in its absorption. Breastmilk has relatively low levels of iron, but the presence of lactoferrin allows it all to be absorbed. Bacteria thrive in iron-rich environments. In comparison, artificial formula milk has five to six times as much iron, but as it is in its free form, far less is available to the infant (formula milk has no lactoferrin). Iron supports the growth of bacteria and raises the risk of gastrointestinal infections. Television ads often promote how "follow-on formula milk" provides more iron for the baby whilst it is developing rapidly. This is often a concern for mothers who can't analyse their breastmilk, and may doubt its quality.

Lactoferrin has several activities that also actively prevent bacterial growth. By binding to iron, it reduces levels available for bacterial growth. It also binds to receptor sites on the surfaces of cell membranes, causing the cells to break down and suppress its viral replication. Most importantly, it helps the cells lining the gut to stop foreign proteins passing through and causing damage. It isn't easily broken down in the gut, and stays intact to be found in the bowel motions of breastfed babies. Only 10% of lactoferrin is saturated with iron, leaving the remaining 90% free to exert its bactericidal (killing of bacteria) activity.

Administration of supplementary iron to a breastfed infant interferes with this level of saturation resulting in decreased bactericidal activity. However, iron supplements given to anaemic breastfeeding mothers do not interfere with the levels of lactoferrin in her breastmilk (Zavaleta, 2005). The concentration of lactoferrin is highest in colostrum and declines gradually over the following 5 months.

Oligosaccharides

Oligosaccharides act to coat the inside of the infant's gut, blocking the attachment of microbes and toxins. Any remaining after this passes on to coat the urinary tract, protecting both from infection. Artificially fed infants have fewer oligosaccharides in their bowel motions, and they are of a different composition to those found in breastfed babies. Although formula-milk manufacturers claim to add oligosaccharides, they have not been proven to have any benefit.

Lysozyme

Lysozyme kills bacteria by causing a breakdown of their cell walls, so that they explode effectively. It also has anti-inflammatory activity. Levels increase during lactation, peaking at around 6 months. It has been suggested that this is to protect the gut during the introduction of weaning foods to the diet. It is found in large concentrations in the bowel motions of breastfed infants, but not those who are artificially fed.

Epidermal Growth Factor

Epidermal growth factor seals the intestine, preventing the absorption of undigested protein, and reducing the risk of allergy. It increases the production of lactase, which breaks down lactose into glucose and galactose. It has been shown (Dvorak et al., 2003) that levels of epidermal growth factor are higher in many mothers who deliver extremely prematurely, compared to those who deliver prematurely, or at term, and that it may be involved in protecting the baby against Neonatal Necrotising Enterocolitis (NEC).

Secretory Immunoglobulin A (IgA)

It is believed that IgA coats the gut, making it impermeable to pathogens, and thereby protecting the baby. Concentrations are particularly high in colostrum. The tight junctions between the alveolar cells are wide open to allow free passage of the immunoglobulins to protect the baby. They gradually close over a few days to protect the baby from other substances, including drugs, getting through to milk.

Anti-inflammatory Molecules

These molecules dampen down the inflammatory reaction to harmful substances (bacteria and virus) in the gut. It may account for the lowered incidence of inflammatory bowel disease in breastfed babies, and the reduction in severity of NEC, whose risk factors include prematurity, formula-feeding, and bacterial colonization. Investigators have identified several growth factors (e.g., Epidermal Growth Factor, Transdermal Growth Factor, Inflammatory Growth

Factor, and other important antimicrobial and anti-inflammatory molecules, including erythropoietin, PUFA, IgA, which are present in breastmilk, but not in formula milk; Frost et al., 2008).

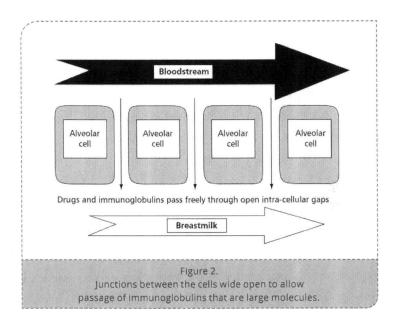

Figure 2.
Junctions between the cells wide open to allow passage of immunoglobulins that are large molecules.

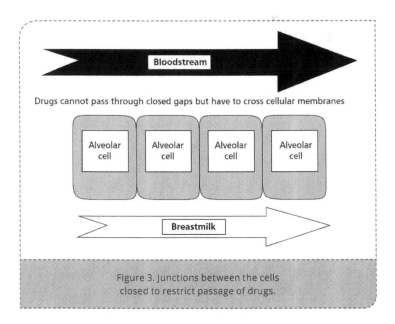

Figure 3. Junctions between the cells closed to restrict passage of drugs.

Bifidus Factor

Bifidus factor promotes the growth of *Lactobacillus bifidus*, which inhibits the growth of harmful bacteria by encouraging an acidic environment, which is less appealing to harmful bacterial growth.

Leukocytes

These white blood cells in breastmilk engulf and destroy harmful bacteria. They are responsible for the longer time that expressed breastmilk can be stored without curdling. Breastmilk can be stored in the fridge for 5 days, whilst formula milk needs to be prepared freshly for each feed.

How do These Factors Protect the Breastfed Infant?

The hundreds of biologically active factors within breastmilk provide protection to the infant against infection and autoimmune reactions. Their presence accounts for the benefits of breastfeeding. Looking at the function of these factors explains why breastfed babies experience fewer gut infections, suffer lower rates of allergic reactions, and absorb the iron in breastmilk more effectively. How amazing is nature, doing all this without us having to think? Why would you not want this for your baby?

To add the final icing to the cake, if Mum is not protecting her baby by breastfeeding, she is increasing her own risk of breast cancer (particularly pre-menopausal; Frost et al., 2008) ovarian cancer, insulin-dependent diabetes, and hip fractures, and she reduces her long-term increases in bone density (Paton et al., 2003; Polatti et al., 1999). Compared to women who have not had babies, those who do not breastfeed have about a 50% increased risk of type 2 diabetes in later life (Liu et al., 2010). *Women who exclusively formula-feed are also more likely to suffer from anemia due to return to menstruation sooner.* Wow, I think you will agree that that is a lot of protection!

Again, I can't stress enough that formula milk has supported many, many babies. If it is your choice, you have my support. It is just impossible to manufacture a "living," continually changing, biological fluid that is individual for every mother. Maybe one day, but not in the foreseeable future. Enjoying your baby is the most important thing. They grow up all too soon!

This chapter may feel very scientific. But I hope you will read it and return to it when you have doubts about carrying on. It contains lots of information on why you, as a family, have chosen to breastfeed your precious new baby.

Take Home Messages

- ◉ Breastmilk contains many factors that are impossible to reproduce and add to formula milk.

- ◉ Formula milk cannot provide protection against infections, and there may be some long-term health conditions because it does not contain these factors.

- ◉ Breastmilk is continually changing to meet the needs of the growing baby, and is the perfect food to nurture and protect your precious baby.

- ◉ Sometimes breastfeeding doesn't work out or is impossible, despite every attempt, and your baby will be well-nourished on formula milk.

Labour and Birth: A New Life Begins!

Labour Day

The day everyone waits for; the day of the baby's birth! There are so many expectations of that day and the final moment of anticipation to see the long-awaited new little person. Most parents now know whether they are expecting

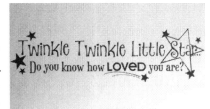

a boy or a girl, and have the clothes, nursery, and accessories all colour coordinated.

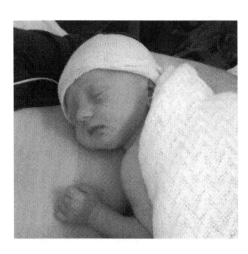

The First Hour After Birth

The first hour after delivery has been called The Golden Hour. During this time, the mother and baby should be left in naked, skin-to-skin contact. This is a time that helps the baby to calm after the trauma of birth, and to adapt to life outside of the uterus. Skin to skin reduces the baby's adrenaline level and settles the heart rate. The mother's body temperature keeps the baby warm, and they need be covered only by a light blanket. In addition, the mother passes on her own natural skin bacteria to provide protection and added immunity, along with antibodies in her breastmilk (Price & Johnson, 2005).

Research that followed 1,250 babies for 3 years from birth showed that skin-to-skin contact with the mother for at least 20 minutes after delivery increased the time for which the mother breastfed by 2.1 months, and that they were exclusive breastfeeding for 1.35 months longer than controls who did not have skin to skin (previous practice) (Mikiel-Kostrya et al., 2002).

The release of oxytocin will stimulate the contractions of the uterus and expulsion of the placenta (Matthiesen et al., 2001). Skin to skin isn't just a nice time to have for cuddling your baby; it has many benefits for the baby, the mother, and breastfeeding.

If, for some reason, the mother is unable to have this first hour with the baby, skin-to-skin contact with dad or grandma would still be beneficial for the baby–and them!

Take Home Messages

◉ In the Golden Hour, the mum and baby should be left in skin-to-skin contact.

◉ If this is not possible because the mum is unwell, can the baby have skin-to-skin contact with Dad or Grandma?

The First Feed

Babies are wide awake in the first hour after birth. After that, they may fall asleep for a period of 2 to 6 hours, during which, it's hard to rouse them to feed.

If left undisturbed on the mother's chest, the baby will usually find the nipple and latch on without help, using the "breast crawl." The mother usually automatically helps the baby to find its way to the nipple with a gentle touch and massage as she explores her new offspring. There is no need for anyone to do anything other than marvel at this beautiful new little person in your lives. By all means, make the mum a cup of tea and a piece of toast (or more). She has worked very hard in the past few hours! It is time for lots of hugs, some phone calls, and celebration.

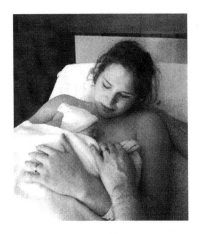

The rooting reflex is automatic. The smell of colostrum is similar to that of uterine fluid. Neonates show preference for breasts covered with amniotic fluid and the odour encourages them to suck. Maternal odours stimulate breastfeeding activity, and the recognition of the mother, and encourages the baby to seek out the nipple (Porter, 2004). There is no need for the breast to be squeezed and pinched, or the baby to be held to the nipple. If we trust in nature, just stand back and wait; the mother and baby will act as one to establish the first feed. So often we rush to weigh the baby and do checks in the haste of a busy postnatal ward, but they could wait or mostly be carried out whilst the baby lies on the mother's chest.

When the infant is peaceful and in skin-to-skin contact with its mother, it will go through nine behavioural phases: birth cry, relaxation, awakening, activity, crawling, resting, and familiarisation, suckling, and sleeping. These result in early optimal self-regulation. Interrupting the process before the baby has completed this sequence, or trying to hurry him through the stages, is counterproductive and detrimental to mother and baby (UNICEF UK Baby Friendly, 2013).

One study videotaped 28 full-term infants immediately after birth (Widstrom et al., 2011). They noted that when the babies stopped crying, they exhibited a short period of relaxation, and then became more and more alert. In this active phase, they moved their limbs, began to root, and look at their mother's face. They then demonstrated a crawling phase, accompanied by noises before licking the areola and finally sucking. Only after this did they fall asleep. The position adopted is frequently termed laid-back breastfeeding, or Biological Nurturing, with the baby laid face down on the mother's body, rather than in her arms (Colson, Meek, & Hawdon, 2008).

What If?

All of the above messages are fantastic if your daughter/daughter-in-law/partner goes into labour normally, at term. But sadly, babies don't always manage to decide to be born in the way or at the time we imagine when we write our birth plans.

What if Your Baby is Born Prematurely?

A baby is premature if born before 37 weeks gestation. There is a wide range of what this may mean for you and your baby, depending on how early he is born. It may mean being admitted to a neonatal intensive care unit (NICU) or special-care baby unit (SCBU), with high-tech interventions to help your baby breathe, maintain temperature, and possibly be fed. It may feel as if the unit "owns" your baby, but this is only because they are working hard to make sure your baby is stable. It is usually seen as important that your daughter/partner is encouraged to provide breastmilk for the baby as it acts as a medicine, as well as nourishment, reducing the risk of the condition neonatal necrotising enterocolitis (NEC), in particular. Breastmilk is easier for preterm stomachs to digest than infant formula milk. It also contains hormones and growth factors that help your baby grow and come home earlier (Boyd et al., 2007). It may be a while before the baby is able to tolerate any feeds by mouth, and has to be maintained on an intravenous drip or a nasogastric tube.

If the baby is well enough to stay with his mother on the post-natal ward, but needs monitoring, you may find that regular heel pricks are taken to check that blood sugars are being maintained at a level that keeps the baby safe. The baby's temperature will also be monitored. Keeping the baby skin to skin will help to stabilize the temperature, whilst frequent feeds will keep the hypogly-caemia at bay. In the early hours after birth, you may find that staff members suggest that some formula milk is necessary until the mum has mastered hand expression and good attachment.

Each individual situation needs to be managed according to the advice of the staff caring for the baby. Even if some formula-milk feeds need to be given, it may be given by cup or syringe, rather than bottle. It does not mean that breastfeeding will not be an option, and it is a good idea to keep putting the baby to the breast as often as possible to stimulate the milk supply. Between feeds, ask for help with hand expression. Any colos-trum you collect can be given to the baby at the next feed.

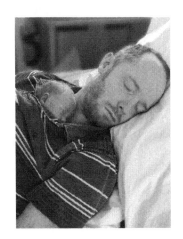

In the times when the mum needs to be away from the baby, like to take a shower or enjoy a meal, there is no reason the baby can't spend time in skin-to-skin time with the dad, as my other son-in-law demonstrated so clearly in this photograph. It is very relaxing and helps bonding!

What if Your Baby is Born by Caesarean Section

If the woman in your life had to have an emergency caesarean section, you, as a family, may have had a tough time in labour. Knowing that she had to have surgery, even if it was under an epidural, rather than a general anaesthetic, is pretty traumatic. Caesarean sections involve surgery. In the first 24 hours after delivery, the new mother may need help to reach the baby in order to breastfeed. She may be drowsy from the pain killers, and so may the baby be. Encourage her to have skin-to-skin contact with the baby when she is awake. When she is asleep, this privilege may be yours. The majority of hospitals now encourage skin to skin in the theatre whilst the wound is sutured (stitched). If it isn't offered, then ask for it. Remember all the reasons it is important.

Many hospitals now allow fathers to stay with their partners throughout the stay in hospital. If this is possible (even if you have to sleep in a chair), your role is to pass the baby to your partner to feed, to change nappies, and of course, to make sure the mum gets regular food and drink. See how invaluable you are? Most of all, this is a time to get to know your new baby and spend time with your partner. Everyone needs lots of hugs!

Mothers who have caesarean sections cannot drive or do any heavy housework for 6 weeks, so your help will continue to be invaluable.

Take Home Messages

- ⊙ Left in skin to skin, most babies will become alert, seek their mother's breast, and self-attach.
- ⊙ There is no need to rush weighing, etc., until after the baby has fed for the first time.
- ⊙ Babies seek colostrum as its odour is similar to that of amniotic fluid.
- ⊙ There is no need for professionals to actively latch the baby on the breast if nature and instinct are allowed to take their course.
- ⊙ Even if the birth didn't go to plan, skin to skin is still important.

THE BASICS OF BREASTFEEDING

Colostrum

Colostrum is the first milk made, often leaked from the breasts in late pregnancy. It is very rich in proteins, antibodies, and immuno-globulins, to protect the baby from the new world he has entered. It coats the gut with protective factors, which form a barrier against foreign substances. The newborn baby gut is very permeable, and colostrum acts as a paint to seal the holes. It also has a gentle laxative effect to clear the gut of meconium. Meconium is the first bowel motion passed by the baby, and is composed of all the materials ingested at the end of pregnancy, and will be discussed under the section about pees and poos below.

Colostrum is thick, sticky, and generally difficult to express using an electric or manual pump (and is lost as it sticks to tubing), but can be expressed onto a teaspoon or collected in a small syringe, using hand expression (see Chapter 7 on expression).

Colostrum is different from mature milk in other ways, as well. It contains more salt, carbohydrate, protein, and less sugar and fat than mature milk. It is only made in small volumes (teaspoon-fuls), which is all that is needed to fill the very small stomach that a newborn baby has. It is the most perfect food for a newborn. Farmers and zookeepers know that a baby animal who is not able to access its mother's colostrum may not develop well. They will often buy colostrum from another animal, if necessary. Colostrum is truly liquid gold to a developing baby in terms of protection and nutrition.

Take Home Message

⦿ Colostrum is made in very small quantities, but it is the perfect first food for a newborn to protect and nourish. It is all a healthy newborn needs.

The Relative Size of a Baby's Stomach

At birth, the capacity of a newborn's stomach is about 7-10 ml, and it is the size of a small marble. By one week, the capacity is about 30 ml, and is the size of a walnut. By one month, it has a capacity of 80 to 150 ml, and is the size of a large egg, or the size of the baby's clenched fist.

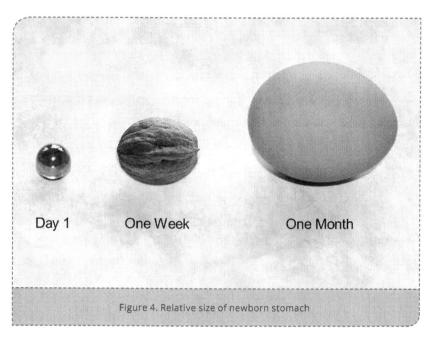

Day 1   One Week   One Month

Figure 4. Relative size of newborn stomach

Babies do not need large volumes of milk. Breastfeeding has the advantage of allowing the baby to stop the feed when he is sated. With artificial feeding, babies are often encouraged to finish the volume of milk being offered, stretching the stomach capacity. It is easy to see, therefore, why formula-feeding can lead to weight gain over and above that which is natural, and therefore, a long-term obesity risk. Often, the first feed of a formula-fed baby will be 30 ml, a considerably larger volume than colostrum will provide.

Take Home Messages

- ◉ The newborn baby's stomach is small.

- ◉ If the baby can't/won't suck, colostrum can be hand expressed onto a teaspoon, which can then be dribbled into the baby's mouth

Mature Milk

Mature milk begins to be produced around the third or fourth day after birth. It increases in volume, and generally appears thinner and whiter (more opaque) in colour than colostrum. You will only see this normally if the mother expresses. It may have a blue tinge to it, or green, or even rusty orange, on some occasions. It doesn't matter. It is perfectly designed to meet the needs of the rapidly growing baby.

In those first few days, it is extremely important to breastfeed at least 8 to 12 times in each 24 hours. The more frequently the breast is stimulated, the more milk is produced. Frequent breast-feeding also helps prevent engorgement (see Chapter 3).

Days after birth	Type of milk produced by breasts	Description
Birth to 2 or 3 days	Colostrum	Thick, yellowish, small amounts
3 to 5 days	Transition milk	Mixture of colostrum and mature milk, more plentiful
5 to 7 days	Mature milk	Thinner, white, plentiful

Table 1. Changes in breastmilk after delivery.

A Diary of Pees and Poos

As the volume of milk increases and changes from colostrum to transitional milk, then mature breastmilk, the baby's stool colour and consistency changes. An exclusively breastfed baby will produce loose and unformed motions of a dark green colour in the first few days. These change gradually to a mustard yellow, sweet-smelling motion. Breastfed babies normally produce frequent bowel motions in the early days. The bowel motions of a breastfed baby are very different to those of a formula-fed baby, which are much more formed and smell less sweet!

Much information can be gleaned from the appearance of the baby's bowel motions (poo).

Lack of stools / infrequent stools in the early days	The baby is not receiving enough milk. This may be due to less-than-perfect attachment. The mother may be experiencing sore nipples. The baby may also be sleepy.
Change to yellow movements from meconium	Milk production has commenced and the baby is feeding well.
Green and frothy movements	The baby is receiving too much lactose. This may be due to an excess of the early less fat-rich milk in a feed, or switching the baby between breasts before emptying one breast first. Green nappies can also be a sign of not enough milk.

Table 2. Changes in infant bowel motions after delivery.

It can be useful to record how many wet and dirty nappies are produced over a 24-hour period to reassure you that breastfeeding is going well. A sheet, such as the one on the following pages, may help. If the baby is not feeding as frequently as the chart suggests, is not wet as frequently, or has not passed a poo, then it may be a sign that help is needed before further problems develop. Babies who don't feed enough can become very sleepy and jaundiced. They sleep so much that they are too good to be true! This can also happen if they are not feeding effectively and accessing their mother's milk. A further sign could be sore nipples for the mother. Some babies can look as if they are feeding well and frequently, but are actually only mouthing the nipple. Poor urine output can be an early sign that help is needed before the baby becomes dehydrated, loses more than 10% of its birth weight, and ends up being re-admitted to hospital.

Meconium

Meconium is composed of materials ingested around the time of birth, and is what gives the first bowel motions the dark, tarry appearance. Meconium is normally stored in the infant's bowels until after birth, but sometimes it is passed into the amniotic fluid before birth, during labour and delivery. The stained amniotic fluid is often a sign that the baby is in some distress, and needs to be delivered urgently. The medical team will suck any out of the baby's mouth or nose immediately after delivery. Sometimes the baby will be admitted to special care for observation in case an infection develops. Colostrum helps the meconium to be passed because it is a natural laxative. Over the first few days, meconium will be replaced by yellow poo, which is an indication that breast-feeding is going well.

The diary below may help you to keep track as to whether your new baby is weeing and pooing with the expected frequency. This may well be something you, the dad, can usefully record to assist.

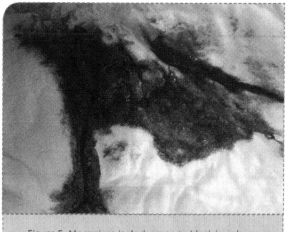

Figure 5. Meconium is dark green to black in colour.

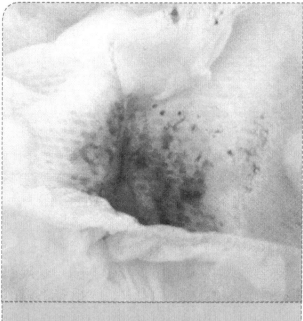

Figure 6. Breastfed baby poo is yellow and sweet smelling.

Day of Birth
- goal to breastfeed 6-8 times -

circle the hour when your baby breastfeeds

midnight   1 2 3 4 5 6   7 8 9 10 11

midday   1 2 3 4 5 6   7 8 9 10 11

tick the W each time your baby has a wet nappy

wet nappies   W

tick the P each time your baby has a dirty nappy

dirty nappies   P

Day 2
- goal to breastfeed 6-8 times -

circle the hour when your baby breastfeeds

midnight   1 2 3 4 5 6   7 8 9 10 11

midday   1 2 3 4 5 6   7 8 9 10 11

tick the W each time your baby has a wet nappy

wet nappies   W   W

tick the P each time your baby has a dirty nappy (expect 2+)

dirty nappies   P   P

Day 3
- goal to breastfeed 8 or more times -

circle the hour when your baby breastfeeds

midnight   1 2 3 4 5 6   7 8 9 10 11

midday   1 2 3 4 5 6   7 8 9 10 11

tick the W each time your baby has a wet nappy

wet nappies   W   W   W

tick the P each time your baby has a dirty nappy (expect 3+)

dirty nappies   P   P   P

Day 4
- goal to breastfeed 8 or more times -

circle the hour when your baby breastfeeds

midnight   1 2 3 4 5 6   7 8 9 10 11

midday   1 2 3 4 5 6   7 8 9 10 11

tick the W each time your baby has a wet nappy

wet nappies   W   W   W   W

tick the P each time your baby has a dirty nappy (expect 4+)

dirty nappies   P   P   P   P

Day 5
- goal to breastfeed 8 or more times -

circle the hour when your baby breastfeeds

midnight   1 2 3 4 5 6   7 8 9 10 11

midday   1 2 3 4 5 6   7 8 9 10 11

tick the W each time your baby has a wet nappy

wet nappies   W   W   W   W   W

tick the P each time your baby has a dirty nappy (expect 5+)

dirty nappies   P   P   P   P   P

Day 6
- goal to breastfeed 8 or more times -

circle the hour when your baby breastfeeds

midnight   1 2 3 4 5 6   7 8 9 10 11

midday   1 2 3 4 5 6   7 8 9 10 11

tick the W each time your baby has a wet nappy

wet nappies   W   W   W   W   W   W

tick the P each time your baby has a dirty nappy (expect 6+)

dirty nappies   P   P   P   P   P   P

Protecting the New Mum and Baby

Just as in labour, you may need to protect the mum from unwanted interventions and unhelpful suggestions. After delivery, there will be some health care professionals and visitors who do not follow the plan you have envisaged, and seem intent on stopping the mum from resting.

So if someone wants to take the baby off to be weighed or examined, just as the mum is about to feed, ask them to wait until the time is more convenient. If the mum is asleep, you may need to prevent people from coming in for a variety of reasons. Maybe it is the cleaner. Of course, standards of hygiene are essential, and of course, the cleaner has a routine. But is it possible that she could delay cleaning your room for half an hour whilst the mum has that longed-for nap? It could be someone who wants to fill in a form, or maybe a support worker that wants to take a blood pressure measurement. If the mum is fit and well, perhaps a delay could be negotiated. Of course, this depends on the health of the mother–if her blood pressure is raised or she has had complications, her health has to be a priority. But in the middle of the night, that doesn't need to involve putting on all the lights! Similarly, if meal time comes around and the mum is breastfeeding, you may need to collect the food for her. If meals get missed, make sure you find a sandwich for her (or whatever she fancies to eat).

Making a Breastfeeding-Friendly Nest

Once home after the birth, you may decide that the mum and baby want to stay in bed for much of the day in the first week: late mornings, an afternoon nap, and early night. Can you make sure that everything she needs is within easy reach? Similarly, if she wants to be up but resting, you can make an area around the comfortable, well-supporting chair. She may need a table for her cup and the plate of healthy snacks that you are making her regularly. It needs to be where she can reach it. Nothing is more frustrating than being able to see the glass of water, but finding it is in the other side of the room. Can she reach her phone? Does she need a charger available? What about the controller for the TV? Does she need painkillers? How about a stool for her feet?

Dad and Grandma, you are in charge of making the mum feel like the most special person in the world, just at this moment. She has produced a beautiful baby for you to adore. She deserves to be spoilt!

Take Home Messages

- ⊙ Make sure the mum is not woken unnecessarily to fit in with hospital routines, which aren't essential to her or the baby's health.

- ⊙ Protect the mum.

- ⊙ Make sure the mum gets food and drinks because breastfeeding makes you incredibly hungry!

- ⊙ Keep telling her she is fantastic.

Settling the Baby

Newborn babies are insecure. They have spent the past 9 months swimming in uterine fluid, contained in a small area, rocked by the body movement of the mother, and hearing her body. After birth, they startle at sudden noises. This is an automatic reflex. They need to know that someone who cares for them is nearby. Skin to skin is the quickest way to settle a baby. They feel the warmth of your skin, they hear your heartbeat, they feel your arms close around them, and this settles them. If the mum is asleep, there is no reason that Dad or Grandma can't cuddle the baby in skin to skin. It is the most relaxing feeling, and allows you time to bond with the baby, to explore the texture of their skin, and to share the rush of oxytocin–the hormone of love.

Some people are adamant that a baby needs routine from day 1, should be put down in a cot from the beginning, and left to self-soothe. I'm really not sure what self-soothe means, but it seems to involve babies being permitted, even expected, to cry themselves to sleep. I will be honest. There is no way on this planet that I could do that. My gut instinct is to keep the baby in close contact to avoid crying. However, there are many books on the market; this is your baby and your choice. I'm hoping that I can empower you to make your own decisions, and throw off advice and comments that don't fit with what you want to do. Hopefully, you three are working as a team and not pulling in different directions. Grandma, they may not be doing what you did, but hopefully you can accept that.

Helping the Mum to Relax

Grandma, you may be able to remember how easy it is to lose confidence in yourself when you have just had a baby. How come everyone else can settle the baby and stop him from crying when you can't? Why does everybody make statements that you interpret as a criticism of your parenting, even if you have only been a parent for 24 hours?

Hormones are changing rapidly. Sleep deprivation and extreme tiredness are beginning to take their toll. Grandmas and dads can help to boost confidence in the new mum. Reassure her that she is doing a good job, that she is a natural mum, and encourage her! She did a great job of pregnancy and birth, of course she can breastfeed, of course she knows what the baby needs, and it is okay to cry for no particular reason!

One of the most important things that you can help her with is relaxing. Oxytocin works in opposition to adrenaline, so the tenser she becomes, the less readily her milk will flow. Her prolactin levels may be high, and she may be making plenty of milk, but not releasing it as quickly as the baby demands. Feeds may become lengthy and tiring, and the baby may be less satisfied if the mum is not having a let-down. Babies also seem to be barometers of a mother's feelings. If she is upset, the baby will usually be crying. The more the baby cries, the tenser the mum becomes. Round and round goes the destructive circle.

How can you help her relax? By making her favourite foods and drinks. Snacks when she is feeding are invaluable. Do you need to take a thermos of hot water up to bed for a midnight drink? Can you pack a box of snacks to keep you both going overnight, Dad? Grandma, can you get up early and make breakfast in bed for the new family? Does she like her neck or feet massaged? Can you look after the baby whilst she has a relaxing bath?

One thing that my daughter and son-in-law found worked for them during feeds in the early hours with a baby who didn't want to settle was for Christian to read their favourite book to her. They chose to re-read their favourite childhood book, *Tales of Brambly Hedge*. It was comforting, simple, had short chapters, and brought back the feeling of coziness of bedtime stories from their own childhood. But it could be anything. I was told that last year, the favourite story for many mums in labour was *Fifty Shades of Grey*!

Being the Gatekeepers

Lots of people want to visit and meet the new baby, and all of you want to show him off. But visits should be short, or else everyone can become very tired. Offers to bring round cake, or a ready-made meal, should be welcomed! People who can do shopping for you are invaluable. All of you around the new mum will also be tired and need to conserve your own energies. You don't have to be Super-Family. People like to help and feel privileged to be asked to undertake a task. We all do. Accepting help is a compliment to their friendship.

Other Reasons a Baby Cries

Babies can cry for reasons other than hunger. As a family, you will very soon become accustomed to the cry your baby makes, and what he is trying to tell you. It may be that he is tired, wants to be held, needs his nappy changed, is too hot or cold, is unwell, or sometimes that he has been overstimulated and needs some quiet skin-to-skin time.

Burping

In the UK, we seem to be rather infatuated with burping babies, feeling that they need a lot of help to bring up wind swallowed during a feed. Usually, if a baby is supported to sit up on the mum, dad, or grandma's lap with an adult hand under the chin, the baby will bring up wind of his own accord. Gently patting the back seems to be an intuitive action. It may be useful to have a cloth under the baby's chin to catch any milk that may be spat up. Alternatively, you can hold the baby against your shoulder to rub the back. This is usually easier once the baby's head control is better.

But What If?

Breastfeeding the Premature Baby in the NICU/SCBU

A discussed in chapter 1, having a baby in NICU or SCBU is very stressful. You may very well feel helpless. You may be stuck in hospital or, worse still, your baby may be in hospital, but the mum has been discharged, and you can only visit hospital. Sometimes the cost of getting to hospital, parking, and eating is expensive, and adds to your stress. Discuss this with the staff, as there may be means of helping you.

However, providing breastmilk for your baby is really important. It is something health care professionals encourage as a medicine, as well as nutrition, because of its amazing protective properties.

Dad, you have a very important role at this time. Your partner may feel very stressed, frightened, and tearful. This is a very scary and unexpected time. You will be needed as a shoulder to cry on almost inevitably. More importantly, you can encourage the mum to express little and often. In order to release breastmilk, it is important for the mother to relax (see the section on oxytocin in Chapter 3). How can you do this? Have photographs of your baby near the breast pump, and encourage your partner to look at them as you talk about how precious your new little one is. A cuddly toy you have specially bought (or one from your own childhood) may help. A relaxing neck and shoulder massage, or foot rub, will also help. Every single drop of breastmilk is worth its weight in gold. Keep encouraging her. You may also need someone to talk to and even cry with. Don't try to be Superman. Be honest about how you feel.

Grandma, you are probably feeling very, very helpless at this stage. You too have a role, which is to be strong for the mum and dad. You may need to take the phone calls from relatives and friends anxious for news. Repeating the same story can be stressful, so you may nominate someone else as a point of contact, or use social media to pass on news. You also can use your nurturing talent by ensuring that the new parents have plenty of nutritious snacks, regular meals, and drinks. Being in a hospital may limit opportunities for fresh and appetizing food (with all due respect to hospital catering).

Hand expressing colostrum initially (colostrum sticks to plastic tubing and the small volumes can be difficult to collect) will provide the baby with all the immunoglobulins and antibodies needed in the first few days. This may be given by syringe, or may be frozen if your baby is too preterm to tolerate it just yet. Remember, the volume of colostrum is measured in teaspoonfuls, but that is all the baby needs.

Soon, the mother will be encouraged to express frequently and regularly, day and night. The milk will provide the perfect start and quantity for when the baby can feed directly. Even before he is able to breastfeed directly, you may be encouraged to have the baby in skin-to-skin contact for prolonged periods, even whilst still attached to tubes. This is called Kangaroo Care.

Usually, you will be provided with an electric pump with which to express. The frequency of expressing needs to be as often as the baby would feed, so pump 8 to 12 times across 24 hours, which must include expressing overnight. I know that it is tempting to sleep through while you can, but this will not help to establish the supply to an optimal level. Milk should be stored in the fridge according to the baby's needs. Extra amounts can be frozen for later use. Breastmilk can be transported to hospital in cool bags with ice blocks, according to the directions of the unit.

Once the baby is strong enough to breastfeed, he may feed directly during the day, when you as a family can be at the unit, but may be bottle-fed overnight. Accommodation overnight may be available, depending on the unit.

It may be traumatic. And there may be times when you are scared for your baby. But there will come a day when you will go home as a family, feeding normally. A time for celebration!

Breastfeeding After a Caesarean Section

It sometimes takes a while to establish breastfeeding after a caesarean section, but it will all come together with patience. Remember that the baby's stomach is only the size of a small marble, and that babies are born with a reserve so that they don't need huge volumes of colostrum, let alone top ups with formula milk. Keep the baby in skin to skin with the mum, and encourage her to feed every time the baby is awake. If the baby has a tendency to fall asleep, make sure he isn't too well wrapped up. Strip the baby, and tickle his hands and feet to encourage suckling.

As with any other surgery, strong painkillers may be necessary during the recovery period. These may leave the mum drowsy, but should not affect the baby. If your partner is taking opiate drugs, such as morphine, she may become constipated. Make sure she eats lots of fruit and vegetables, and drinks watery drinks. She may need laxatives, which you can buy or have prescribed (see chapter 8). A breastfeeding pillow or a cushion may be useful to protect the scar from contact with the baby.

Within a few days, the scar should heal, mobility should improve, and apart from the mum not driving, you will be like any other family.

What can Dads and Grandmas do in the first few days after the baby is born?

- Make sure that the mum has plenty to drink. She may be very thirsty, so make sure she can reach a drink when she is breastfeeding. She may need a straw. Watery drinks are ideal, but try to avoid too many caffeinated, fizzy drinks (because they aren't healthy), or too much strong coffee or tea, which may make her jittery.

- Make sure that the mum has plenty of healthy snacks available between meals. Breastfeeding (and birth) can leave you hungry. It can be tempting to eat chocolate, cake, and biscuits. They are great for treats, but fruit is ideal so the mum doesn't get constipated.

- Keep an eye on the breastfeeding log. Is the baby feeding frequently enough?

- Change the nappies, and fill in the poo and wee log!

- Encourage mum to get as much rest as she can. Being available to the baby 24 hours a day is exhausting.

- Consider whether you need to nap as well, if you are going to be awake to help the mum overnight.

- Make sure there aren't too many visitors. It is lovely to show off your wonderful new baby, but it is also tiring.

- If visitors have coughs and colds (or other bugs), ask them to stay away. You have enough to deal with in the first few weeks without preventable illness!

- Do the housework, washing, ironing, and shopping.

- Cuddle the mum and baby.

How to Get Breastfeeding Basics Right

If I had one message to get to every new family planning on breast-feeding their baby, it would be "get the attachment right," and offer a feed whenever the baby is awake, and you are on the way to success. If there is pain for more than a few seconds, then you need to seek help urgently. It does take time to get accustomed to the feeding of breastfeeding. A baby's suck is, relatively speaking, three times stronger than that of an adult's. I'm not asking for personal information, but that isn't a suck we are used to, multiple times a day.

Positioning and Attachment

The words "positioning" and "attachment" have, in the past, been used together. They are inextricably linked, but also different. Positioning is more about the way that the mother is sitting or lying, and how she therefore brings the baby to the breast. Since most of us spend the majority of our feeding sitting up, we can start there, and move on to reclining and feeding while lying down.

Positioning

The mother needs to be in a chair that is comfortable, but also provides good support to her back so she can maintain an erect, but relaxed position, however long the feed lasts. Chairs with arms can be a problem, as they be just at the height where we want the baby to be, so the mum may need to sit in the middle of a sofa or in an armless chair, such as a computer chair. The height of the chair is important too. The mother needs to have her feet flat to make a lap for the baby to lie in. Often, it is more comfortable to have the feet raised, for example, on a stool, or a pile of books, or the baby's chair. Whatever works for her, her height, and your furniture.

Many mothers now buy breastfeeding pillows on which to support the baby. These are expensive and may not meet the needs of the mother. My daughter bought the most popular version in the USA, but it proved to be too thick and brought the baby too high. It also didn't "sit" around her waist. We found other uses for it. It made a great back support and later, a support for tummy time, and sitting up for the baby. Another brand had a strap which held it in place. It also provided a flatter surface, which worked for her. However, it was only used for a brief period of time before being abandoned as unnecessary!

So looking, in general, the mother' needs to be comfortable enough to maintain the position for as long as the feed takes.

- She needs to be relaxed and not forcing her body to hold a pose that is unnatural.
- Arms should be in line with the body, with elbows tucked into the side rather than sticking out at an odd angle.
- Lean back into the chair, and do not lean forward.
- The baby should be brought up to the breast, not the breast dangled down towards the baby.
- The lap should be flat to support the baby with feet raised as necessary.
- Shoulders need to be relaxed and dropped into a comfortable position.

When we are tense, the first thing that happens is that shoulders are raised and the head sinks down into them. One really useful thing that Dad or Grandma can do is to watch the mum, and remind her of the way she is sitting. A shoulder and neck massage can be really useful in supporting the breastfeeding mother. It only takes a few minutes, but can help the let down and give the mother confidence. It also feels great for you to be useful, and most pleasurable for the mum!

Some mothers find it easiest to have the baby on their chest with themselves in a laid- back position at about 45 degrees. This allows the baby to self-attach, as it may have happened at the first feed.

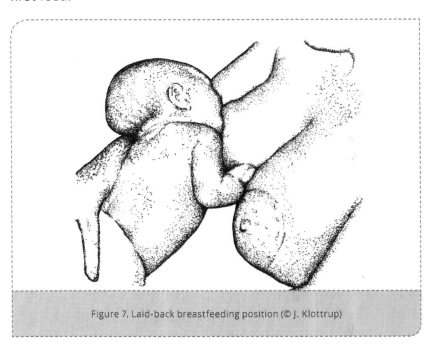

Figure 7. Laid-back breastfeeding position (© J. Klottrup)

As breastfeeding continues, the mum will often want to master breastfeeding when laying down. Although it is frequently recom- mended that babies are not allowed to co-sleep with their mother for fear of smothering or laying on the baby, over 75% of breastfed babies spend at least part of the night in their parent's bed. It increases the prevalence of breastfeeding. In one study, it was found that breastfeeding was significantly higher among the groups that shared beds constantly, or early, for each of the first 15 months after birth (Blair et al., 2010). There is further information on the UNICEF Baby-Friendly website (www.unicef.org.uk/BabyFriendly/ News-and-Research/Research/Bed-sharing-and-infant-sleep/). ISIS has detailed fact sheets on safe sleeping (www.isisonline.org.uk/).

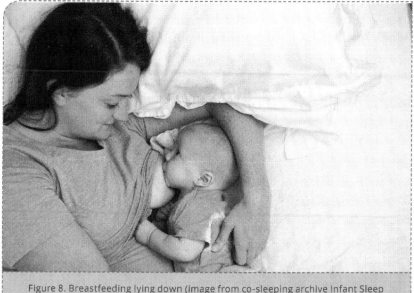

Figure 8. Breastfeeding lying down (image from co-sleeping archive Infant Sleep Information Source, www.isisonline.org.uk courtesy of Rob Mank)

As mothers, we automatically sleep with the baby in line with the breast, the lower arm above our head, and knees raised to form a nest where it's impossible to roll onto the baby, and the baby is away from pillows, but has ready access to the breast.

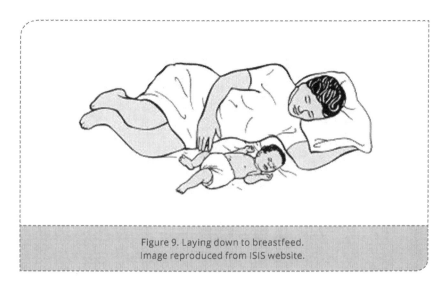

Figure 9. Laying down to breastfeed.
Image reproduced from ISIS website.

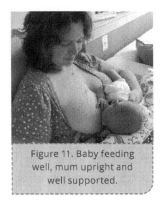

Figure 10. The rugby hold (©Juliet Klottrup).

Some mothers find the "rugby hold" easier to achieve. This is where the baby is held alongside the mum, rather than across her tummy. In exactly the same way the baby's head needs to be in a straight line with the body, head free to move and, the body gently supported along the arm.

For breastfeeding, we need the baby's belly towards the mum's belly, facing the food. If the mother has nipples that point outwards, or very pendulous breasts, we may need to adjust the position so that the baby is facing the nipple. No two breasts are the same and we are all individuals – here, shape and size do not matter.

Figure 11. Baby feeding well, mum upright and well supported.

Take Home Messages

- Make sure that the mum is sitting comfortably with her back supported and her feet flat on the floor or a stool.

- Some people find special breastfeeding pillows useful. You can also manage with a normal pillow/cushion, or by lying back slightly at about 45 degrees.

- The mum needs to be comfortable for however long the feed takes.

- Don't forget drinks, snacks, phone, and TV remote in easy reach.

Attachment

Attachment is the way that the baby is latched onto the mother's breast. This is a vital part of effective breastfeeding. If the attachment isn't quite right, the baby will not be able to access all of the milk. If attachment is not 100%, the baby may be restless, hungry, and not gain weight whilst the mum may experience damaged nipples, frustration, and may feel she has no option but to give up breastfeeding. The important factors to look out for when the mum is bringing the baby to the breast are:

- The baby's body should be in a straight line with the whole body facing the food (nipple and breast). If the baby is laid flat on the mum's lap, he will have to turn his neck at right angles to the shoulders. If you try drinking a glass of water like that, you will soon discover how uncomfortable and difficult this is. The baby needs to be facing in towards the mum.

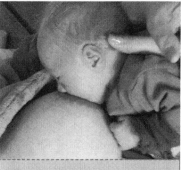

Figure 12. Baby in good position for breastfeeding, head in line with body and head free to move.

- Lying on their backs with the belly upwards is the position we use to bottle-feed a baby. When we bottle-feed a baby, we often lay the baby flat on his back, but still with the head and body in line. If you have never watched a baby being breastfeed, this may seem to be the natural way to hold a baby.

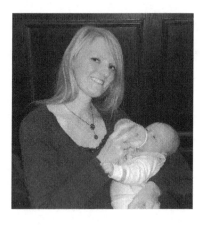

- Make sure the mum supports the neck, shoulders, and back so that the baby can tilt his head back easily. If the baby is held around the head, there is an automatic response to pull the head back. Also, if you press forward on the back of the head to encourage the baby to go onto the breast, it is more likely to push the chin down onto the chest, making it difficult to swallow. Finally, it wouldn't be impossible to think that many babies may have a headache after the delivery, and further pressure on the head is likely to be uncomfortable

- Remind the mum to move the baby from her cleavage out towards the nipple rather than starting with the baby's mouth opposite the nipple. This encourages the baby to bring the lower lip in first and take a big mouthful of breast tissue.

- Sometimes it helps to pull the baby's bottom in close to the mum's belly, which tilts the head back, leaving the mouth clear. Babies all have snub noses and nostrils slightly further apart than an adult's to enable them to breathe, even if their nose appears to be buried in the breast. They don't suffocate. If they can't breathe, they will let go of the nipple.

- It is probably easier for you than the mum to see that the baby's lower lip and chin is in contact with the breast first, with the top lip than curling up over the breast tissue to make a good seal.

- When the baby is correctly attached, you will be able to see the baby's jaw moving (rather than the cheeks), and often, the tops of the ears move as the full movement spreads. You will also be able to hear long rhythmical sucks and swallows interspersed with fluttery sucks as the baby rests.

- The baby should come off the breast by itself looking slightly drunk, relaxed, and well-satisfied. You may see milk dribbling from the mouth. But it doesn't matter if you don't.

- The mum should not be experiencing pain to breastfeed. It may be temporarily a bit uncomfortable (stretchy, stingy, odd) when the baby latches, as a baby's suck relative for its size is three times stronger than an adult's.

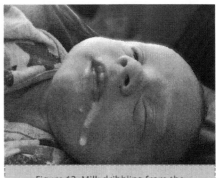

Figure 13. Milk dribbling from the baby's mouth as he comes away from the breast satiated.

Signs That the Baby is Not Well-Attached

1. Baby's mouth not wide open and lips curled inward.
2. Only the nipple or a small amount of breast tissue taken into the mouth.
3. A clicking noise can be heard during the feed.
4. You don't hear regular, deep swallows.
5. Mother experiences unrelenting pain during the feed.

Baby-Feeding Cues

Early breastfeeding cues are:

⊙ Moving of the head from side to side as the baby searches for the breast. Sometimes they will bob around so much that they will move themselves into a perfect breastfeeding position.

⊙ Moving the tongue around, and often sticking it out.

⊙ Putting hands to the mouth, sucking anything that is nearby.

⊙ Wriggling and squeaking.

My grandson was adept at always keeping his hands close to his mouth, a position we had seen him in on his pregnancy scans. We had to find means of holding his hands gently away so that we could get him to attach. Some people choose to swaddle the baby, but then that misses the lovely feeling as the baby strokes and kneads the breast during a breastfeed, just like kittens and puppies do. This is a means of encouraging the let down too. Allowing the baby to find his own way to the breast often results in more successful attachments than trying to force him on. Nature does know best sometimes!

Sore Nipples

Nipples can be very easily damaged in the first few days after delivery if the baby's attachment is not perfect. This is incredibly painful and can be soul destroying. If something hurts, why would you voluntarily keep doing it many times a day for the good of someone else? As an onlooker, the desire to remove the pain is enormous. It is really hard to watch someone you love be in pain. But when it relates to pain on breastfeeding how do we, as Dad and Grandma, help? The worst thing we can do is to say,

Ah yes, I heard breastfeeding was painful. I think it gets better or maybe your nipples just toughen up.

Well, if you gave the baby a bottle, it would give your nipples a rest and then maybe they would heal.

Not helpful! Instead, it's completely demotivating and likely to end in tears. The mum knows why she chose to breastfeed. It is about her health and that of the baby. She's trying really hard, but she hasn't done this before. Just like getting into the car for the first time. There will be a few grated gear changes or stalling of the engine. What the mum needs is the equivalent of a driving instructor coaching her along and encouraging her that she is doing a great job.

So the first thing we need to go back to is the mum's position (see above). Is she sitting upright and with her back supported? Some modern sofas are not helpful, as they encourage us to slouch down with a curved back. The old-fashioned nursing chairs were hard-backed and low. Is it possible to find something similar in your house? Maybe a computer chair, or even a dining chair. Are her feet flat on the floor, or slightly raised to make a flat lap? If she is anticipating pain, her shoulders will be raised up to her neck: a neck massage and a comforting hug will help.

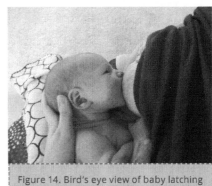

Figure 14. Bird's eye view of baby latching well at the breast.

Then we look at this wonderful new baby. Is he laying with his head and body in a line, facing in towards his mum, back supported, but head free to move? Are his hands in the way? Can you hold them gently, but lovingly away until he is latched onto the breast without getting in the way? Encourage the mum to have him in the centre of her body, then to move him outwards towards her nipple so that he comes in towards the breast with his chin making contact well below the nipple first and scooping up onto the breast as he opens his mouth wide. If he isn't opening his mouth wide, tease him by touching the nipple to the top and bottom lip, and wait for him to open wide. If you miss the moment, hang on; he will do it again.

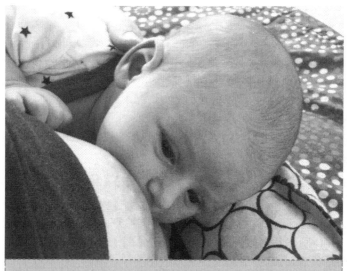

Figure 15. Photograph shows baby facing the breast, head free to move, body tucked into mum so nose free. Relaxed and pain-free breastfeed.

Remind the mum to bring the baby up to the breast, not lean over the baby, or she will get backache. Once the baby is attached, she can lean back, tuck his bottom into her, and relax. What you should see is that the baby's nose is free of the breast, his hands are relaxed, and he is tucked in with his neck free to extend.

If, after this, the feed is painful for more than the first couple of seconds, then you need to phone a friend. This could be the midwife, a local volunteer, the national helplines, a lactation consultant, or a friend who has been there. The mum needs to be able to feed without excruciatingly sore nipples, and avoid any damage to the nipples.

But What If?

If There is Damage to the Nipples

If there is more than just a graze, apply a simple product into the crack to stop it from drying out. If the nipple develops a crack, it may very well scab over. At each feed, the scab will be removed by the baby's suction, or even as the breast pad is removed where it has stuck. This makes the wound open up again and deepen. The moisturiser stops the scab forming and helps the crack to heal from the bottom up. This is called "moist wound healing." The product you use does not have to be a special, expensive product aimed at breastfeeding mothers. A simple, white, soft paraffin will do the job adequately.

There is no evidence that any cream applied to nipples to prevent cracks is effective. Nipple damage is caused by a less-than-perfect attachment, and a cream can't stop that.

Take Home Messages

- ⊙ Sore nipples are not an inevitable part of breast-feeding.

- ⊙ If nipples do become sore, look again at the mum's position and the baby's attachment.

- ⊙ Understand the mum's discomfort, but keep encouraging her.

- ⊙ If the pain continues, get help.

- ⊙ Suggesting a bottle is not helping!

Grandma, you may remember that we were taught to dry our nipples if we developed cracks. This would have encouraged scab formation, but at least prevented nipples from becoming soggy, which also prevents healing. Think of leaving a cut covered with a Plaster for more than a few days. The skin becomes too soft to heal. There was also an aerosol product that was supposed to prevent damage, and anesthetise the nipple as well. This was just an antiseptic in a spray, and made the nipple taste horrible. I can't bear to think of what it must have done to my children's taste buds! Just like the creams marketed today, it wasn't a magic wand.

One Breast or Two?

The well-attached baby should be allowed to breastfeed from the first breast for as long as you can see he is sucking and swallowing. In the early days, if the baby does not come off the breast, this is a good time to use breast compression. When breastfeeding well, the baby should let go of the breast, as described above. The second breast can then be offered, and the baby may or may not continue to feed. The next feed should commence on the last side to be used. Some mothers wear bracelets to remind themselves which side that was, while others put safety pins on the bra straps or tie a ribbon. These are not necessary, as it is usually possible to feel which the more "full" side is.

Breast Compression

Breast compression is a way of encouraging the milk to flow, even when the baby has stopped or slowed down the sucking. It can be useful when the baby is tired or drowsy, for instance, if jaundiced. It can also encourage milk consumption if the baby's weight gain is not as fast as we would like. It can be invaluable if the baby is spending a lot of time on the breast, but not actively sucking. It may not be something you need to use, but it can be a very useful tool to have in your mental cupboard of magic.

Breaking Suction

If the baby is not well-attached and is causing pain, it can be necessary to break the suction to take the baby off the breast. This is done by inserting a clean finger into the corner of the baby's mouth, and pressing the lips apart above the nipple. This sounds easy, but a baby's suck is very strong, and to take him off the breast may not be easy as his natural instinct is to hold on tight.

Breast Compression Described by Dr. Jack Newman

- Hold the baby with one arm.

- Support your breast with the other hand, encircling it by placing your thumb on one side of the breast (thumb on the upper side of the breast is easiest), your other fingers on the other, close to the chest wall.

- Watch for the baby's drinking, (see videos at nbci.ca), though there is no need to be obsessive about catching every suck. The baby gets substantial amounts of milk when he is drinking with an "open mouth wide—pause—then close mouth" type of suck.

- When the baby is nibbling at the breast and no longer drinking with the "open mouth wide—pause—then close mouth" type of suck, compress the breast to increase the internal pressure of the whole breast. Do not roll your fingers along the breast toward the baby. Just squeeze and hold. Not so hard that it hurts, and try not to change the shape of the areola (the darker part of the breast near the baby's mouth). With the compression, the baby should start drinking again with the "open mouth wide—pause—then close mouth" type of suck. Use compression while the baby is sucking, but not drinking!

- Keep the pressure up until the baby is just sucking without drinking, even with the compression, and then release the pressure. Release the pressure if baby stops sucking, or if the baby goes back to sucking without drinking. Often the baby will stop sucking altogether when the pressure is released, but will start again shortly as milk starts to flow again. If the baby does not stop sucking with the release of pressure, wait a short time before compressing again.

- The reason for releasing the pressure is to allow your hand to rest, and to allow milk to start flowing to the baby again. The baby, if he stops sucking when you release the pressure, will start sucking again when he starts to taste milk.

- When the baby starts sucking again, he may drink ("open mouth wide—pause—then close mouth" type of suck). If not, compress again as above.

- Continue on the first side until the baby does not drink even with the compression. You should allow the baby to stay on the side for a short time longer, as you may occasionally get another let-down reflex (milk-ejection reflex), and the baby will start drinking again, on his own. If the baby no longer drinks, however, allow him to come off or take him off the breast.

- If the baby wants more, offer the other side and repeat the process.

- You may wish, unless you have sore nipples, to switch sides back and forth in this way several times.

- Work on improving the baby's latch.

- Remember, compress as the baby sucks, but does not drink. Wait for the baby to initiate the sucking. It is best not to compress while the baby has stopped sucking altogether.

Ways to Tell if a Baby is Well-Attached

- The mum experiences no pain during the feed.
- The baby comes off the breast by itself, and looks relaxed and satisfied.
- The baby's arm should be relaxed.
- The baby's body in a straight line, turned in to the mum's belly.
- The baby should have the mouth wide open with more of the areola (darker area) visible above the nipple than below.
- You can hear long rhythmic swallows interspersed with some rests.
- You can see the whole jaw move, not just the cheeks going in and out.
- The baby's lips are flanged outwards.
- The baby has much of the areola in his/her mouth (depending on size), but with more on the chin side of the breast.
- The chin is pressed into the breast with the nipple just touching or clear of the breast.
- The baby's bottom is tucked closely into the mum.
- There is no need to work hard at burping.
- Taking the baby off the breast may be necessary, but not easy.

But What If?

Engorgement

As the milk comes in, there is an increase in blood supply to the breast. Around the third day after delivery, the breasts become larger and can feel hot, sore, and heavy. It is important at this stage to keep on feeding frequently, making sure that the attachment is as good as possible. Sometimes it is necessary to hand express a small amount of milk to keep the breast soft enough for the baby to be able to latch on. A technique called reverse pressure softening can also help. If the breast is too full, the nipple can appear to be less protractile and harder for the baby to take a full mouthful of. Some mothers can have a low temperature, feel achy, miserable, and tearful. With regular emptying, the symptoms should be minimised and last no more than 12 to 24 hours.

It can also help to use warm compresses on the breast, or have a shower briefly before the feeding, to encourage milk flow, and cold compresses after the feed to help with feelings of bruising. Cold cabbage leaves in the bra can also be helpful. This is not just an old wives' tale, but actually has a limited evidence base (Nikodem et al., 1998). One hundred and twenty women, 72 hours after delivery, were randomly allocated to have normal care, or to apply cabbage leaves. The study group was more likely to be exclusively breastfeeding at 6 weeks, and to breastfeed for longer. The effect may have been due to the cabbage leaves, or just being part of a study, which provides an increased self-esteem.

Gentle breast compressions and massages during the feed can also help drainage.

Day 3 is often the really hard day when mums need lots of encouragement and reminders about why breastfeeding was the way you chose to feed the baby and why. Look back at the poster at the beginning!

Reverse Pressure Softening

When the breast is very full of milk, this technique can help to relieve the pain and swelling, as well as helping the baby to latch on more effectively. See diagrams below.

The aim is to make the area just behind the nipple soft enough to help the baby latch on easily. It is important to be very gentle with handling the breasts when they are full of milk to avoid bruising or producing blocked ducts. Firmly, but gently press on the areola at the base of the nipple. Press inwards towards the chest area using the flat side of both thumbs above and below the nipple. Continue to press around the nipple, one small area at a time. An alternate method is to curve the fingers like a flower where the mouth of the baby would be, and press in slowly and gently. As the swelling is pushed back away from the nipple, the areola is softened, making it easier for the baby to get a big mouthful of breast tissue. The fluid within the tissues is moved back into the lymphatic system. The let-down may also be stimulated, producing a flow of milk from the nipple.

This may be something which you can encourage the mum to do, reminding her of the technique when she is very full or maybe if you are both comfortable with it, you can very gently do this for her.

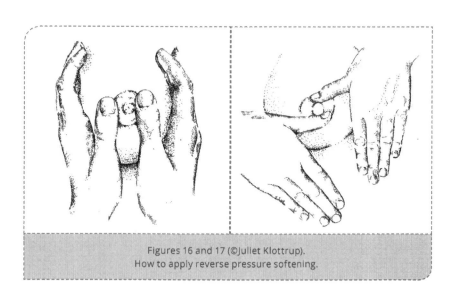

Figures 16 and 17 (©Juliet Klottrup).
How to apply reverse pressure softening.

Neonatal Jaundice

It is very common for babies to develop jaundice 2 to 3 days after birth. In the womb, the baby has excess red blood cells to help to absorb all the oxygen needed. Once born, these are not needed by the baby, so they are broken down and release an excess of bilirubin. Babies' livers are not fully functioning, and it takes a little while to do this. The levels of bilirubin in the blood are monitored by blood tests, as well as watching the degree of "sun-tan" the baby shows to observant eye of the midwifery/obstetric team. Bilirubin is excreted in wee and poo. Colostrum is a natural laxative, so the more that a baby feeds, the more bilirubin will be removed from the body. If the symptoms persist, the baby will become drowsy, and not feed as frequently, so producing a vicious circle. Jaundiced babies need to be encouraged to feed effectively 8 to 12 times a day. If the mother experiences pain, it is important that she gets help as soon as possible. Apart from causing agony, sore nipples are a sign that the baby will not be accessing as much milk as the mum is making, which will not help jaundice. It is sometimes advised to place the baby in front of a sunny window, weather permitting.

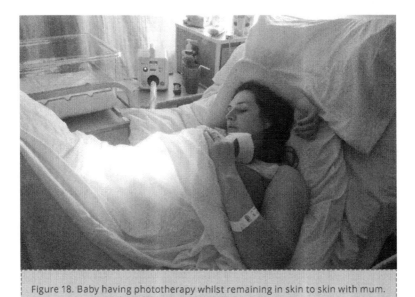

Figure 18. Baby having phototherapy whilst remaining in skin to skin with mum.

Ongoing high levels may need treatment. It usually means that the baby is placed under ultraviolet lights to help with the breakdown. This, in turn, makes the baby slightly dehydrated, so additional breastfeeds may be needed. There is no need for formula milk or water if the baby is feeding well. In fact, these can be positively unhelpful and discouraging to the mum. High bilirubin levels can be harmful to the baby's brain and other organs so they should not be ignored. Bili blankets can be placed onto the baby whilst he is still in skin-to-skin contact, although he will need to have his eyes protected.

Jaundice usually resolves by around the end of the first week.

Breastmilk jaundice is a less common form. It begins when the baby is around 2 weeks of age. Its cause is not well understood. It occurs in babies who are alert, feeding well, weeing, and pooing as normal, and gaining weight. It can last for around 6 weeks, but doesn't need treatment if the baby is fit, well, and term. However, it may need to be investigated. It is probably caused by factors in the breastmilk that block certain proteins in the liver that break down bilirubin. Breastmilk jaundice tends to run in families. It occurs equally, often in males and females, and affects 0.5% to 2.4% of all newborns.

Take Home Messages

- ⊙ It is common for the baby to appear suntanned around the second or third day after birth.

- ⊙ Encourage the mum to breastfeed 8 to 12 times a day.

- ⊙ Make sure the mum gets help to optimise her milk supply.

Words of Encouragement

Is everyone feeling daunted at this point, thinking how does anyone ever manage to breastfeed without pain and without problems? All these hiccups will not happen to you, I'm sure. I want you to have somewhere to go to if there are problems, and a way out to solve the problems without thinking you need to give artificial formula milk supplements, or give up, unless you choose to do so. Breastfeeding is no longer seen as "easy," as it was even 50 years ago, because bottle-feeding has become the norm. Dolls and toys come with bottles, and we have a society that has been less than breastfeeding-friendly for many years.

It has fascinated me, over my past 30 years of breastfeeding support, that some people breastfeed against all the odds, overcoming challenges day after day, week after week, but persevering. Others give up relatively quickly and happily. Is this linked with the support available to them? Is this about bottle-feeding being the norm in their family and social group? There are exceptions to every rule. The choice is yours. I can only give you information and options in supporting your feeding journey with this baby. What I can say is that breastfeeding can be totally simple and easy. However, it can be complex and challenging. Through my Facebook page, *Breastfeeding and Medication*, or my website www.breastfeeding-and-medication.co.uk, I am happy to do my best to support you on your journey.

The Science of How Breastfeeding Works

If we understand how breastfeeding works, it is often easier to understand why things can go wrong, and how we can stop it from getting worse, but best of all, fix it. So bear with me. I'll try not to make it too complicated! Think of it as like understanding the offside rule, or a new recipe you have watched chefs effortlessly prepare on TV.

Anatomy of the Lactating Breast

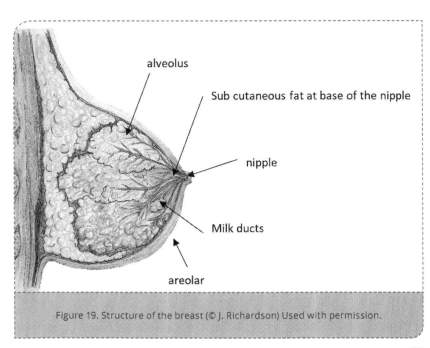

Figure 19. Structure of the breast (© J. Richardson) Used with permission.

In 1840, Sir Astley Cooper produced diagrams based on dissections of the breasts of lactating mothers by pouring hot wax down the milk ducts before eroding the surrounding skin and tissues, leaving a wax model of the duct system. Until 2005, this was the only study of the anatomy of the breastfeeding breast until an Australian team investigated the system of ducts more closely using sophisticated ultrasound technology (Ramsay et al., 2005).

The size and shape of the breast, nipple, and areola vary dramatically between women. This does not affect the ability to breastfeed, nor does the size of the breast itself, which is determined by the fat tissue. Most women have one breast larger than the other, with the left often being the largest

The Areola

The areola is the circular pigmented area around the nipple. It turns a darker, reddish brown during pregnancy, and retains the colour subsequently. However, the colour varies with the general complexion. Montgomery tubercules are small sebaceous glands present in the areola. They become enlarged in pregnancy, and appear as small pimples. They are believed to secrete a lubricating substance during pregnancy and lactation to protect the nipple from bacterial infection. Too frequent washing may remove this protection, and may also make the skin drier with the nipple and areola becoming more prone to soreness and cracking.

Nipples

The nipples usually become more erect in pregnancy and in breastfeeding, as does their ability to stretch. Babies breastfeed. They do not nipple feed. They form a "teat" from the surrounding areola tissue, and not just the nipple.

But What If?

Inverted Nipples

In a small proportion of women, the nipple is inverted (goes inwards), rather than erect, or it becomes inverted when the areola is gently compressed. Whilst the skin becomes more elastic during the third trimester of pregnancy in preparation for nursing, some of the cells in the nipple and areola may stay attached. Some nipples don't protrude when stimulated, but can be pulled out manually. The severely inverted nipple responds by disappearing completely inwards. Exercises to pull out the nipple, and a device to draw them out using a pump, have been recommended in the past, but have not been shown to help in studies. If your partner has inverted nipples, it is probably best to talk to a breastfeeding expert locally before your baby is born to help with how to attach the baby. It should not affect your partner's ability to breastfeed, and they could possibly just need a bit more help. Remember, if there is pain during feeding, or the baby does not appear to be getting enough milk, phone a friendly breastfeeding expert.

Breastmilk supply is controlled by two hormones: prolactin, which makes the milk, and oxytocin, which causes the ducts to constrict and release breastmilk.

Prolactin

- ◉ Levels of prolactin start to increase in late pregnancy.

- ◉ Production of breastmilk is held in check by the levels of oestrogen and progesterone, which drop dramatically at delivery.

- ◉ Stimulation of the nipple by suckling causes the production of prolactin. Even mothers who have not given birth to a baby can produce breastmilk by such stimulation.

- ◉ If there is no nipple stimulation because the mother chooses not to breastfeed, prolactin levels continue to fall.

- ◉ Mothers who smoke are reported to have lower prolactin levels (Baron, 1986).

- ◉ Beer is reported to increase prolactin (DeRosa, 1981).

If the baby dies before birth, the milk production may still commence. For some mothers, this can be a heart breaking reminder that there is no baby. For others, it has been found to be comforting to donate the milk to special care babies (Welborn, 2012).

Oxytocin

When a baby feeds at the breast, oxytocin is released from a centre in the brain within one minute. It quickly enters the blood stream, and causes cells within the breast to contract and expel the milk. This is known as the milk ejection reflex (MER), or "let down."

The release of oxytocin can also be triggered by the thought of feeding the baby, visualising the baby, smelling something that reminds you of the baby, or hearing the baby cry. Sometimes mothers will begin to release and leak milk in anticipation of a feed. If this is at an inconvenient moment, pressing the heel of the hand against the nipple can stop the leak. If this happens frequently, she may need to wear breast pads. Most mothers do.

Some women report a tingling sensation in their breasts that happens just before milk begins to drip. Others notice a stronger let down with sharp needle-like pains. Still others are unaware of any sensation. The release of milk does not rely on what the mother feels, nor does lack of sensation does not imply poor let down or supply.

Oxytocin also causes the uterus to contract, which helps to control postnatal bleeding and a more rapid return of the uterus to the pre-pregnant state. The cramps may be experienced as period-like pains at each feed during the first few days after delivery. These become more pronounced after each delivery, and a mother who has had more than one baby may need to take regular painkillers in anticipation of this discomfort. The uterus continues to contract for 20 minutes after feeds finish, although secretion of oxytocin returns to normal levels 6 minutes after the nipple stimulation ceases.

Let-down can be *temporarily* inhibited by embarrassment, pain, tension, fatigue, or anxiety: all sensations associated with adrenaline release. Milk continues to be produced under the influence of prolactin, but ejection is slower, and may cause the baby to pull away from the breast in frustration. Relaxation will help the let-down.

For new mothers, this is most apparent if trying to feed somewhere you feel uncomfortable. When she needs to breastfeed in public, try to go with her or encourage her to take someone she trusts with her. Dad or Grandma, you can sit close to the mum, and keep talking

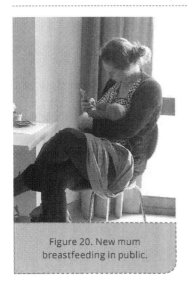

Figure 20. New mum breastfeeding in public.

normally. Your reassuring presence is really helpful. Despite all the stories in the media, complaints about mothers breastfeeding in public are rare, and against the law in both the UK and most states in the U.S. Carry a soft scarf to drape over her breast, or use the baby's blanket. Usually, the only sign that a baby is being breastfed is not the sight of the mother's naked breast, but the way she looks down at her baby to check that all is well!

Take Home Messages

- ⊙ Prolactin release begins after delivery, whether or not a woman intends to breastfeed.

- ⊙ Frequent feeds increase the prolactin level and therefore, the milk supply.

- ⊙ Oxytocin helps the milk to be released from the breast.

- ⊙ It can be temporarily inhibited by fear, pain, or embarrassment.

- ⊙ The womb contracts in response to oxytocin. This can be painful, and may require mum to take regular painkillers.

- ⊙ Oxytocin is shared in a loving, supportive environment.

Oxytocin has also been called the hormone of love. It is released when we stroke an animal, when we have positive social interactions (e.g., in a supportive group, and when we touch one another with love by cuddling, caressing, or making love). It is also known to reduce stress. It increases trust and reduces fear, and, most importantly, facilitates bonding. It's a hormone we need and enjoy, whether we know it or not. When I go to work with a group of breastfeeding mothers, I come away feeling relaxed. Cuddling my grandson to sleep leaves me dreamy and happy. Oxytocin is magic!

Feedback Inhibitor of Lactation

The production of breastmilk is governed by the removal of breast-milk from the breast. It would seem logical that if you notice that if you express after 4 hours, you get more milk than after 2. However, that only works for a short space of time. If milk is left to accumulate in the breast, it triggers a protein to be released: feedback inhibitor of lactation (FIL). This has a negative effect on milk production, so the less milk that is removed from the breast, the less milk is made. Poor milk removal can be caused by infrequent feeds, less-than-perfect attachment, use of supplementary bottles of formula milk, use of a dummy to delay feeds, and missing feeding cues.

Take Home Messages

- ◉ You can't store milk in the breast.
- ◉ The more the baby breastfeeds, the more milk you make.
- ◉ Breasts can never be completely emptied, and milk is made as the baby feeds.

CHALLENGES TO BREASTFEEDING

Conditions affecting the baby, which may impact breastfeeding, vary in the number of babies they affect. I hope this chapter is not information that you need, and that your baby's breastfeeding journey is smooth, but just in case ...

Fussy Babies: The Evening Period, Often Called "the Arsenic Hour"

This is the time just when you want to relax, get the evening meal, or watch TV, and the baby decides to fuss–maybe cry, maybe feed incessantly. It is frustrating to parents who may finally be spending some quality time with their offspring to find them to be very unhappy little people.

This is a time when we have in the past diagnosed "colic." We have assumed that pulling legs up to chests, and crying is a sign of pain. It isn't necessarily so. This is the only way babies under about 4 months have of showing their feelings. It just means "I'm upset." Sadly, the arsenic hour comes just when we are at our most tired. What was the good time of the day has become a trial to get through.

Babies will often cluster feed during the evening to stock up their energy for longer sleep periods overnight (perhaps, if you are really lucky!). They may not sleep for more than about 10 minutes, so you may have to learn to eat one-handed, or take it in turns. Convenience foods, or meals cooked earlier in the day, may become a necessity. Dad, have you watched any of the TV cooking programmes now so much in vogue? Fancy trying out a new recipe to treat the mum? Or maybe you could take the baby for a bath and playtime while she cooks? There are lots of things that two pairs of hands can do that one pair, with a baby on the hip, can't. Grandma, could you provide some food cooked and chilled for the parents to warm up later? While we need quick food, ideally, we still need healthy food!

The other factor that may help, in my experience, is to make sure that the mum eats well at breakfast and lunchtime and, if at all possible, has a short nap as this seems to maintain the energy levels.

What many women fear is that they have run out of milk in the evenings. As the baby feed more, the breasts never get to feel that they have "filled up," and she may describe herself physically and emotionally as wrung out. Breasts can never be totally emptied— she may not be able to express any breastmilk—but it will be produced in response to the baby's sucking stimulation. Each time he feeds, he puts in an order for more milk to be available.

What is your job, Dad and Grandma? Encouragement, reassurance, and maybe playing with the baby is most useful. Using a dummy on the baby may produce peace and quiet for a short time, but misses out on an opportunity to stimulate milk, so use judiciously.

Frequent Feeding

How many drinks, snacks, and meals have you had in the last 24 hours? Breastmilk provides all of those to babies. Some feeds will be long, and the baby may sleep for a long period afterwards, just like we may do after a large meal. At other times, they may snack frequently for short periods. I have to admit that I often do that in the evenings! Sometimes it is very frequent and short feeds, which may be particularly true in hot weather to quench thirst. So if the baby has just fed, and then 20 minutes later, she wants more, maybe she just wants some more dessert, or a cup of tea.

Sometimes babies cluster feed in the evening, just before bedtime in order to stock up on calories before a longer sleep. You don't need to count the times a baby feeds in 24 hours, as long as it's above the minimum in the first few days. Just watch the wees and poos. Trust your partner/daughter's body and the baby's instinct.

If, however, despite feeding frequently, the baby is not putting on weight or weeing/pooing, then phone a friendly breastfeeding expert, particularly if feeding is painful.

Biting

Everybody assumes that a baby who has teeth will bite his mother when he is breastfeeding, and therefore, teeth will bring an end to breastfeeding. This is not, in fact, the case. Babies move their tongue over their lower gums in order to breastfeed. Occasionally, and more often when they are teething, babies will bite. If you apply a teething gel or liquid onto the gums before the feed, this often removes the baby's need to bite down on anything that is in their mouth, be it a teething ring or a nipple. It is often a mother's natural instinct to shout out when the baby bites, as it really hurts. It may be down to you to remind the mum that this isn't a deliberate ploy to hurt her, and that the baby really didn't mean it (this may need to be repeated as she grits her teeth).

Taking the baby off the breast with a firm, but gentle "no" will soon let the baby get used to the idea that biting means the milk is removed for a few moments. It often occurs at the beginning or end of a feed, often when the mum is not paying full attention to what is happening, so beware. This stage will not last after the tooth has come through, I promise, but the teething period does go on for quite a while.

For some mothers, there can be a soreness around this time not related to biting, but to a change in the acidity of the baby's saliva. Rinsing the nipples with a solution of one teaspoonful of bicarbonate of soda in a pint of water after feeds can help. This pain has, in my experience, often been diagnosed as the first symptom of thrush.

If the baby has actually cut the base of the nipple when biting (as my own daughter did when she was 10 months old), treating it as any other wound and applying a smear of moisturiser to heal from the base will help if it is deep. It is very painful, so Dad and Grandma should be very sympathetic, remind the mum that it will be okay, and doesn't mean the end of breastfeeding.

Other Reasons for Biting

Some babies also use this as a means of signalling frustration that the milk flow has slowed down, or that the mum is not paying them any attention. What is also more likely at the end of a breastfeed is that the baby is playing. If the mum knows her flow is slow, for whatever reason at that time, maybe you could massage her shoulders or feet to help her relax, or bring her a drink. Above all, don't panic. Just go back to basics of positioning and attachment, skin to skin, and chill out.

Growth Spurts: 6-Week Crisis!

Historically, we have talked about babies having growth spurts: periods when they suddenly want to feed more frequently, leaving the mum feeling drained and exhausted. There does seem to be times when this happens, and it is often around 2 weeks, 6 weeks, and 3 months. Surprisingly, there is no research that shows that during these periods, the baby's growth is increasing.

At 6 weeks, in particular, just when you think everything to do with breastfeeding is settling down, your baby turns into a hysterical, unsettled, screaming, red-faced bundle of anger. Your partner may lose all confidence in her ability to produce enough breastmilk. Friends and relatives may comment that, obviously, the milk has dried up, or isn't good enough for the baby. The mum may find herself feeding so frequently that it feels like she hasn't gotten out of the chair all day, and her nipples are sore from constant feeding. Just for 24 to 48 hours, life will grind to a halt whist the baby wants to feed constantly.

Trust me, it will pass if you follow your baby's cues. He is feeding frequently to increase the milk production (although milk consumption doesn't vary that considerably over the first 6 months). Many families feel tempted to offer formula milk bottles at this time in desperation to get the baby to settle. Remember what we said about prolactin? The more the baby feeds, the more milk is made. If you give a feed of formula milk, the breasts may actually lower the supply if the baby then misses a feed (feedback inhibitor of lactation). Milk cannot be stored in the breast. I am not saying you can never give formula milk at this time: it is your baby. However, hopefully this information will provide you with the confidence to keep going. Exclusive breastfeeding for 6 months is our gold standard to protect the baby long term.

If we follow your baby's feeding cues, then we will notice feeding periods will vary within the day, from day to day and week to week. With confidence that frequent feeding will result in more milk being made, we may moan about the baby being demanding or irritable, but we all rejoice in how much our baby is growing, so actually, it is positive! I might not phrase it quite like that to a tired mum who has been feeding the baby every 1 to 2 hours overnight, again! What we know is that if you respond to your baby, and give extra attention (e.g., more breastfeeds) for a few days and probably nights, the fussy period (feeding frenzies) seems to pass. So growth spurts, or fussy periods, or whatever we call them, are not a cause for concern: just a normal phase every baby goes through. Breastmilk has not suddenly become of poor quality or decreased in volume. The message is "trust in your body, darling. Can I make you a sandwich and a cup of tea?"

Is the Baby Getting Enough Milk?

Because breasts don't come with a gauge showing how much milk has been taken it is easy to worry how much the baby has taken. "Is my baby getting enough milk?" is one of the commonest questions new mothers ask. Fear that they aren't taking enough is one of the commonest reasons given for stopping breastfeeding at all stages of feeding.

So how can you tell if the baby is getting enough breastmilk? If the baby is:

- ⊙ Feeding frequently,
- ⊙ Has a deep latch with periods of sucking interspersed with fluttery rests,
- ⊙ You can hear swallowing,
- ⊙ He has the right number of wet and dirty nappies for his age,
- ⊙ He is calm and relaxed after feeds, and
- ⊙ He is gaining weight.

Then he is having enough milk. He should also have periods of being awake and alert during the day without being hungry.

	Total	Duration of breastfeeding				
	%	<2 w	2-6w	6w-4m	4-6m	> 6m
Engorgement	36	20	28	33	45	46
Worry about having enough milk	35	29	40	44	43	32
Baby having difficulty taking the breast / not sucking effectively	21	31	30	24	19	14
Blocked milk ducts	14	4	10	12	16	18
Mastitis	12	5	11	11	15	15
Thrush	8	2	7	10	7	9
Tongue-tie	5	4	6	5	4	5
Abscess	1	1	1	2	2	1

Table 3. Problems experienced by breastfeeding mothers at varying stages of lactation. Data from Infant Feeding Survey (2010).

It is normal for babies to lose weight after birth. They are born with extra fat stores to sustain them until the mother's milk comes in. They may lose up to 10% of their birth weight, but if they are not pooing and weeing as expected (see diary of wees and poos), this needs to be investigated and a breastfeed observed by someone skilled at assessing attachment sooner rather than later. Babies should regain their birthweight within the first 10 to 12 days after birth, and gain approximately 1 oz per day until they are around 3 months of age.

How to Tell if Your Baby Really Isn't Getting Enough Milk

In babies between 10 days and 4 weeks, if the baby is:

- Sleeping for more than 4 hours at least once in a 24-hour period,
- Not producing at least 6 wet nappies a day,
- Has pink uric acid crystals visible in the nappies,
- Not producing a minimum of one mustard yellow poo a day,
- Crossing 2 centiles on the weight chart, and
- Not alert and playful at least once in 24 hours.

It can also be a problem if the mum is experiencing painful nipples throughout every feed. These are signs that you need help with attachment first and foremost. The vast majority of mothers can produce enough breastmilk to satisfy their babies. However, sometimes "advice" to feed on a schedule, to restrict duration of breastfeeds, excessive use of a dummy, failure to respond to early feeding cues, or to accept that breastfeeding hurts will have an effect on milk transfer. Milk remaining in the breast passes a message back via FIL that more than enough is being made and to reduce supply. A vicious circle then starts.

If the baby is given formula milk, and he sucks it all, that will further confirm to the mother that she doesn't have enough milk and/or it isn't good enough, further eroding her confidence. This is not necessarily true. Milk from a bottle is easy to access, and babies will suck most things put in their mouth. Try your clean finger and see what happens.

If the mother wants to change her baby onto formula milk, or to supplement, I'm not attempting to make you or her feel that that is wrong. This is her baby and her life, but I hope this book enables you, as a family, to make an informed choice. By the way, if you do choose to go down that route, there is no difference between any of the brands of milk, despite their advertising claims. The content of formula milk is carefully controlled, and any additional ingredient proven to have benefits would be required to be added to all brands.

So if you think the baby is really not getting enough milk, it is important to get someone to help as soon as possible. There are a variety of drop-in groups around the country, and you should have been told about them before leaving the maternity unit.

Up to 14 days, you can call the midwifery unit and discuss your concerns with a midwife. After this period, you should have the contact detail for the mother's health visitor. Although doctors are wonderful (and I can't praise them enough), they do not have much training on breastfeeding support and problem-solving techniques, unless they have a specific interest. Nor do they have time to watch your daughter/partner feed. This inevitably leads the problem to become a medical one, and you may be offered medication, or have formula milk suggested. If you feel your baby is unwell, then naturally, they should be the first port of call, and you may need to have the baby admitted to a paediatric ward for monitoring and support. Don't panic; this should be supportive, and may help you all relax to get 24-hour-a-day help, especially if you all left hospital very early after the baby's birth.

While you find help, make sure that the mum is feeding as frequently as possible—at least every 2 hours—and is kept in skin-to-skin contact with one of you (but is taken to the mum to feed as soon as he is awake). All of you try to rest as much as possible, but make sure the mum gets lots of meals, snacks, and drinks, ideally taken to her in bed while she rests.

Conditions Affecting the Baby That Impact Breastfeeding

Tongue-Tie

A baby needs to be able to use his tongue to be able to remove milk from the breast well. If the tongue is anchored to the floor of the mouth, the baby cannot do this effectively so he is not able to access all the milk his mother is producing, and she is likely to suffer nipple damage.

There are many signs that tongue-tie is causing problems with breastfeeding:

⦿ Nipple pain and damage,

- The nipple looks flattened after breastfeeding,

- You can see a stripe on the nipple at the end of a breastfeed,

- The baby keeps losing suction while feeding, comes on and off, and sucks in air,

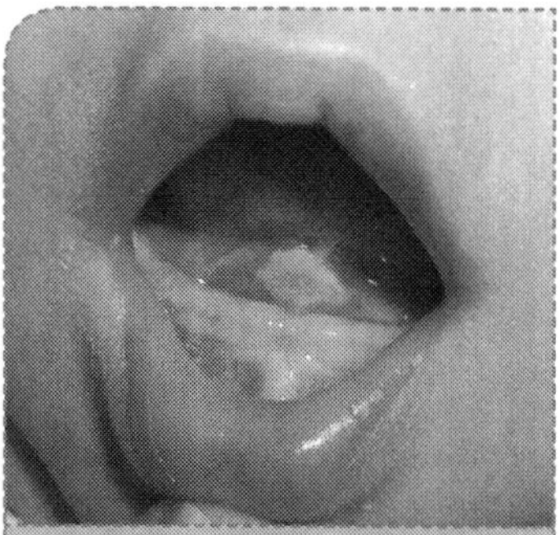

Figure 21. Picture of tongue tie in a baby. ©Carolyn Westcott. *Reproduced with permission*

- The baby makes a clicking sound when feeding,

- The baby fails to gain weight,

- The baby cannot poke his tongue out beyond his gum or lips, nor move sideways, and

- The tip of his tongue may be heart-shaped, or may look flat or square instead of pointed.

Tongue-tie is more common in boys than girls, and there is often a family history. It is said to be present in up to 10% of babies. Were you breastfed, Dad? Can you stick your tongue out? Grandma, does the pain bring back memories for you?

Even if the front of the tongue is free to move, sometimes there is a posterior tongue-tie, where a small amount of tissue still prevents the tongue moving effectively and stops breastfeeding from becoming pain free. It often cannot be seen as abnormal, but identified by an expert feeling under the tongue with a gloved finger. Don't try this yourself!

Where tongue-ties cause feeding difficulties, snipping of the frenulum (the skin under the tongue, can be carried out painlessly, without sedation or local anesthesia, using a blunt-ended pair of scissors). It can have an instant effect, helping the mum to pain-free breastfeeding straight away, or it can take a few days. It appears sore, but apparently does not concern the baby. Access to services varies across the UK and USA, and some people end up paying specialists to snip the tongue-tie (Ballard, Auer, &

Khoury, 2002; Geddes et al., 2008; Griffiths, 2004; Hogan et al., 2005; Tongue-tie.org.uk).

In Australia, 24 babies were studied before and after the tongue-tie division (Geddes et al., 2008). After the procedure, the latch improved in all babies, and they all were able to take more milk from the breast with less pain.

The National Institute of Health and Clinical excellence (NICE, 2005) issued guidance that there are no major safety concerns about division of tongue-tie, and confirmed that there is some evidence to suggest that it can improve breastfeeding.

Colic

Colic is probably every parent's nightmare. We all hear horror stories as to how miserable it makes evenings with a baby! Grandma, did your babies have it? I know my eldest did, and it wasn't fun.

Colic has been defined as "spasmodic contraction of smooth muscle causing pain and discomfort." In studies, it has been defined as lasting 3 hours a day on more than 3 days a week, for at least 3 weeks (Wessel et al., 1954). Symptoms are usually described as high-pitched, inconsolable crying accompanied by flushing of the face, drawing up of the legs, passing wind, and difficulty in passing bowel motions (Barr, 1951).

The cause of colic remains a mystery. Four possible causes have been suggested (Lucassen et al., 1998):

1. Problems within the gut caused by a cow's milk allergy, lactose intolerance, or excess wind.
2. A behavioural problem.
3. Excessive crying at the extreme end of normal.
4. It is a collection of symptoms difficult to explain (that helps a lot!).

In most babies, symptoms resolve by 3 to 5 months of age, but the period can be very exhausting. Symptoms are often worse in the evenings. Up to 25% of babies show symptoms. It is more common in formula-fed babies, and those whose parents smoke are twice as likely to experience symptoms of colic as those who don't (Balon, 1997).

Medication is often used to treat colic. The research behind these is not that extensive, and every baby has "magic wands" that work for them. No one product works for every baby. Suggested approaches include:

- Simethicone drops (Trade names *Dentinox©, Infacol©*). These are believed to bind bubbles of wind. One study concluded that simeticone is no more effective than a placebo in the treatment of colic, although it may be perceived as so by parents (Metcalf et al., 1994).

- Lactase drops (Trade name Colief®). Expressed "fore-milk" should be mixed with the drops and left during the feed, and then given to the baby at the end of the feed to be effective, according to research (Kanabar et al., 2001).

- Eliminating cow's-milk protein from the diet can be effective in treating babies with suspected cow's-milk-protein allergy (CMPA). In breastfed babies, this entails the mother removing all dairy products from her diet. Permanent dietary restrictions should not be undertaken without professional support and guidance. Changing the mother's diet to this extent means not just avoiding obvious dairy products, like milk, yoghurt, and cheese, but most convenience foods, cakes, biscuits, chocolate, etc. If a breastfed baby is thought to have CMPA, the mother should eliminate all sources of cow's milk from her own diet as well as that of her baby for a minimum of 3 weeks. Although improvement may be seen after 3 days, it may not resolve for 4 weeks (Ludman et al., 2013).

Feeding with artificial formula milk in the first 4 to 6 months of life increases the risk to the cow's-milk-protein allergy compared to exclusive breastfeeding (Vandenplas et al., 2007). Just 0.5% of exclusively breastfed infants show reactions to cow's-milk protein compared to 2% to 7.5% of formula-fed infants.

For further information, see the fact sheet on Cow's-Milk-Protein Allergy that I have written for the Breastfeeding Network.

www.breastfeedingnetwork.org.uk/wp-content/dibm/cmpa-nov14.pdf.

Alternatives for colic solutions, which work for some babies, are carrying around, possibly in a sling, driving around the area in a car, or placing the baby near white noise (e.g., a washing machine).

Reflux

Many babies spit up milk. Dr. Jack Newman has described it as "a laundry problem, not a medical problem." However, it causes so much distress to parents. It is really difficult to know how much milk a baby has thrown back up. Do they need more now? Was this a sign that they were over full, so they don't need more? We all worry about babies bringing back milk, but in all likelihood, the baby will just look at you, completely unconcerned.

Reflux happens when the contents of the baby's stomach rise into the gullet (oesophagus). The sphincter muscles at the top of the baby's stomach tend to be weak. You only need to worry if the baby spits up so much that he does not gain weight, or seems distressed. Friends will have given you lots of outfits, so I'm sure you will have plenty of changes of clothes. Don't forget to take at least one set out with you (for the mum and baby, and maybe even you, Dad), and have plenty of bibs, tissues, or wipes around.

If you are worried, then go and see the doctor who may prescribe medication for the baby. Gaviscon® is the most commonly used medicine. These medications do tend to cause some constipation, and are fiddly to give to a breastfed baby, as the contents of the sachets have to be mixed with water or expressed milk, and fed to the baby part way through a feed, which is not always easy. In the U.S., Gaviscon is usually in the form of drops, which are usually easier to give to the baby. There are other alternatives that also cut down the acidity of the gut (e.g., ranitidine and omeprazole liquids), which your GP may prescribe.

Conditions Relating to Breastmilk Itself Causing Breastfeeding Problems

Lactose Overload

Babies whose mothers have a plentiful milk supply may suffer from lactose (the sugar in breastmilk) overload. These are babies who cannot seem to drink all that the mother produces, so the breasts may still feel uncomfortable after even a long, effective feed. As a result, the babies consume a lot of the earlier milk, which has a relatively more plentiful amount of lactose. This passes through the baby more quickly, and can result in poo that is green, frothy, and frequent. He may also have a nappy rash. The baby's weight gain may be more than adequate, but he may appear to be hungry, unsettled, and often very windy. This commonly leads to a very confused mum.

Thinking back to the wee and poo chart from the days after the birth, what hasn't gone in, can't come out, so frequent wee and plentiful poo means that the baby is getting enough. But maybe we need to do something to help the baby be more settled.

In many cases, discussing the latch and improving the attachment a bit can resolve problems as the baby is finally able to empty the breast properly.

Cow's-Milk-Protein Allergy

Anecdotally, more and more mothers are deciding (or being advised) that their child is demonstrating a cow's-milk-protein allergy or intolerance (CMPA). Colic is one example, as previously discussed. Symptoms that may indicate CMPA can affect many organs (see Table below). Feeding with formula milk in the first 4 to 6 months of life increases the risk to cow's-milk-protein allergy (CMPA) compared to exclusive breastfeeding (Vandenplas et al., 2007). Only 0.5% of exclusively breastfed infants show reactions to cow's-milk protein compared to 2% to 7.5% of formula-fed infants.

Where CMPA is suspected in a breastfed baby, the recommended treatment is for the mother to remove all sources of products containing cow's milk from her diet, ideally under medical supervision. This includes not just obvious dairy products like butter and cheese, but ones that are hidden in convenience foods. Mothers should be prescribed a supplement of two tablets of 1,000 mg of calcium, and 10 micrograms of vitamin D (400 IU) every day. Where solid foods have been introduced, all sources of products containing cow's milk should also be removed from the baby's diet. In some cases, children may also be allergic to soya protein, and if symptoms do not resolve this, it should also be removed from the mother's diet. It will usually take between 2 and 4 weeks for symptoms to disappear. It is suggested that milk is then reintroduced to ensure that this has been the cause of the symptoms (Ludman et al., 2013; NICE, 2011).

Organ Involved	Symptoms
Gastrointestinal tract	Frequent regurgitation
	Vomiting or diarrhoea
	Constipation (with/without perianal rash)
	Blood in stool
	Iron-deficiency anaemia
Skin	Atopic dermatitis
	Swelling of lips or eyelids (angio-edema)
	Urticaria unrelated to acute infections, drug intake, or other causes
Respiratory tract (unrelated to infection)	Runny nose, otitis media
	Chronic cough or wheezing
General	Persistent distress or colic (wailing/irritable for ≥3 h per day) at least 3 days/week over a period of >3 weeks

Table 4. Symptoms of cow's-milk-protein allergy in babies (developed from VandenPlas, 2007).

Where a diagnosis of CMPA is confirmed, the mother should avoid cow's-milk products in her diet for as long as she is breastfeeding. She will continue to require support to manage her nutrition, particularly where the elimination diet is over an extended period of time. A dietician or other health care professional managing the case will recommend which point reintroduction of cow's milk should be trialled, and how this should be managed. Care should also be taken with the weaning diet, and appropriate alternative sources of calcium included for the baby under the supervision of a dietician. There is generally no need to add special prescription formula milk if the mother is breastfeeding.

Lactose Intolerance

Lactose is the sugar in breastmilk. The amount of lactose in breast-milk is independent of the mother's consumption of lactose, and hardly varies. However, the quantity of lactase, the enzyme needed to breakdown the sugar, does vary. Lactose intolerance occurs when the amount of lactase (the enzyme) is insufficient to break-down the lactose (the sugar) and enable absorption. The production of lactase begins to decline from the age of 2 years, and most adults are lactose intolerant to some degree.

Lactose intolerance often gets blamed for symptoms like colic. Primary lactose intolerance is a rare, inherited metabolic disorder. A truly lactose-intolerant baby would fail to thrive from birth, and show obvious symptoms of malabsorption and dehydration. In Finland, the gene for congenital lactase deficiency is relatively common. Researchers identified 16 cases of congenital lactase deficiency over 17 years (Savilahti et al., 1983). In each case the mother reported watery diarrhoea, usually after the first breastfeed, but up to 10 days after birth. By the time lactose intolerance was confirmed, all infants were dehydrated, and 15 of the 16 weighed less than at birth. On a lactose-free diet the children all caught up with their growth.

Some premature babies are temporarily lactose intolerant due to their immaturity. Babies can also be temporarily lactose intolerant (secondary lactose intolerance) after gut infections, which damage the surface of the villae in the gut (where lactase is produced). This can also happen after a mother has taken anti-biotics. However, no treatment is necessary, nor change in milk, and the symptoms will resolve in a relatively short space of time.

Lactase Drops

Addition of lactase enzymes (Colief®) to breastmilk has been suggested as a treatment for colic and lactose intolerance (Kanabar et al., 2001). Formula milk, or expressed "fore-milk," had lactase or a placebo added, and incubated for a period before being given to the baby. Formula milk was refrigerated for 4 hours, and then re-warmed. "Fore-milk" was incubated during the feed, and given at the end of the feed. The total crying time over the 10-day treatment period was reduced in all 46 infants, and in the 32 "compliant" families, it was statistical significantly reduced. Lack of compliance (undefined) was possibly due to a high proportion of non-native English speakers. It is expensive and rarely that effective. Help with improving attachment, to enable the baby to drain the breast more effectively, is usually more effective.

Soy Formula

Soy formula milk is often suggested if symptoms of lactose intolerance are suspected. This should not be given to babies under 6 months due to the high content of plant oestrogen. The sugar in soya milk is glucose, which is also more likely to cause dental decay (CMO update, 2007).

Conditions Affecting the Mother That Can Impact Breastfeeding

Blocked Ducts

A blocked duct can occur at virtually any stage in breastfeeding: from the early days until the first year and beyond. A blocked duct is an area on the breast where milk has leaked out into the breast tissue behind a kink in a duct. These kinks can be caused by a knock or pressure on an area, which is full of milk. It could be after lying on a pajama button, having a play fight with a toddler, or wearing a tight-fitting bra. It is important to drain the area of milk frequently. An analogy is a hosepipe that has been stuck in the shed all winter and has been bent. When you come to use it again in the spring, it may split behind the bend, and spray water out behind.

The symptoms of a blocked duct are a dull ache over an area which may feel lumpy and appear red. It may rapidly develop into feeling fluey and achy with a headache.

Symptoms resolve with frequent feeding and/or expressing. Hot compresses on the area to encourage the milk flow helps. Anecdotally holding an electric toothbrush against the area helps to break up the blockage. It is important to encourage the milk flow, but not to attempt to squeeze the site, as this causes bruising and the risk of cellulitis.

Mastitis

Mastitis is an inflammation of the breast, and rarely an infection. It can develop from a blocked duct that hasn't been resolved, or may appear without warning. Many health care professionals automatically prescribe antibiotics, and most online discussion forums suggest that these are necessary to cleat symptoms quickly. In the light of public health concerns of over use and resistance to antibiotics, they are best avoided unless self-help measures have failed to relieve symptoms over a 24-hour period.

Symptoms of mastitis are a hot, red area on the breast, which is painful. It is usually accompanied by a raised temperature, and more severe aches and pains, like a flu virus. Initially, it is very similar to a blocked duct, but more intense. The mother may also feel depressed and weepy. Inflammation and depression are often associated.

Self-help measures, just as for a blocked duct, are to keep that breast as empty as possible, as frequently as possible. If the baby is unwilling or unavailable to breastfeed, this may necessitate expressing. Gentle pressure is essential to prevent further damage from bruising. Stroking across the area with the nail side of the finger rather than the finger pad can be useful. Applying warmth, either by soaking in the bath, shower, dry heat in the form of a heat pad, or hot water bottle, encourages milk flow. As for a blocked duct, holding an electric toothbrush against the area appears to help.

Since mastitis is an inflammation, it often responds well to taking ibuprofen rather than Paracetamol. Back in 1995, it was first suggested that antibiotics may help to resolve symptoms of mastitis by their anti-inflammatory activity, rather than antibacterial (Inch & Fisher, 1995). Ibuprofen relieves temperature, pain, and inflammation, whilst Paracetamol has no anti-inflammatory activity. Both drugs can be taken together in full dose to relieve symptoms.

Mastitis affects up to 30% of mothers at some stage during breastfeeding. Most commonly, it is seen around 6 weeks after birth, or during the period when babies go longer between feeds or sleep for longer overnight. It can often happen unexpectedly after a day out (e.g., a wedding).

It may be that you, Dad or Grandma, may be the first to put together the bigger picture of the mother feeling fluish, achy, and tired, while complaining about sore breasts even before the red area is obvious. Remind her to keep feeding, and get her some painkillers and fluids.

When should you see your doctor or midwife? If symptoms of mastitis do not begin to resolve after 24 hours of frequent feeds, or her temperature stays high, then it may be advisable to consult a doctor for antibiotics alongside frequent feedings as well. Antibiotics usually given are flucloxacillin, cephalexin, or erythromycin (WHO, 2000).These are all safe to take during breastfeeding, although they can lead to very loose and runny poo, sometimes with colicky pains in the baby too. Although the mother may feel poorly and discouraged, this is not the time to stop breastfeeding suddenly, nor to take notice of anyone who suggests that the antibiotics are not suitable for use in breastfeeding. Keep encouraging and supporting her.

If your partner or daughter is diagnosed with mastitis that does not clear up with two courses of antibiotics and frequent feeding, make sure that she is sent for an ultrasound to check for the possibility of an abscess, and that the milk is cultured to see which antibiotic is needed to kill the infection (Dixon & Khan, 2011).

Breast Abscess

A breast abscess is a very rare complication in breastfeeding. It can happen out of the blue, or it can happen if the mastitis was badly managed. It is associated with an infection where the body lays down a capsule around the infection. It needs antibiotics immediately, and often for the area is drained of the pus. This may be via a syringe placed carefully into the abscess by a surgeon using ultrasound to direct the needle, or it may need surgery to drain it, leaving an open wound. It is very rare, but needs to be treated urgently.

The skin over an abscess often has a pitted orange-peel appearance. Despite the seriousness, it may not be painful.

There is no reason to stop breastfeeding if the mother develops an abscess. If any of the pus gets into the breastmilk, it will make some babies vomit it back, while others will not react. The baby will not contract an infection via breastmilk. Some people believe that while milk is leaking where it has been drained, the wound will not heal. This is not true, and, in fact, factors in the breastmilk help to prevent further infection. It can be very worrying, though, as the milk will leak out each time the baby feeds, or as the let-down occurs on the other side. Pressing an absorbent pad of gauze can help to keep the area dry. If the wound is too close to the nipple, it may mean that the mum has to express on that side for a while.

Thrush on the Nipple

Anecdotally, nipple thrush is something that many mothers hear about from their friends, and dread. It produces agonising pain in the nipples after feeds, which goes on for up to an hour. I have written several information leaflets for the Breastfeeding Network over the past 15 years, first to highlight the existence of this condition, and later to try to convince everyone that thrush is not responsible for all breast pain.

The symptoms of thrush in the mother are:

⊙ pain-free latch and breastfeeds, but agonising pain after the feed is over,

⊙ no change in colour or shape of the nipple after feeds,

⊙ pain in both nipples/breasts,

⊙ pain the same after every feed, and

- a positive swab of the nipple cultured for fungal and bacterial infection.

The symptoms of thrush in the baby are:

- white tongue with plaques that do not wipe off,

- a positive swab of the mouth cultured for fungal infection, and

- pulling away from the nipple without letting go. This can also be due to less-than-perfect latching, and frustration from not getting access to all the milk.

It is important to ask the doctor or nurse to take the swabs to confirm the growth of thrush, as it is often difficult to be sure that this is the cause rather than a less-than-perfect latch, bacterial infection, white spot, Raynaud's, or pain as a result of undiagnosed tongue-tie.

Treatment of confirmed thrush is:

- miconazole oral gel (Dakarin®) applied a small amount at a time to all parts of the baby's mouth using a clean finger, and

- miconazole cream (Dakarin®) applied sparingly to the mother's nipples after every feed.

If symptoms still have not resolved, then oral fluconazole tablets may be prescribed for the mum in case the infection has spread into the ducts. This should be avoided in babies less than 6 weeks of age unless thrush is definitely confirmed by swabs because the drug can make the baby sick and suffer severe stomach pains. In young babies, the pain is far more common, due to less-than-perfect attachment.

White Spot on the Nipple

White spot is a blocked outlet on the surface of the nipple behind which milk accumulates. Pain is helped if the overgrowth of skin is removed either by gentle rubbing following soaking in warm water, or by using a sterile needle. Mothers usually describe pain is as like a pinpoint, and they point to it exactly with one finger. It is advisable to ask a health care professional to remove it with a sterile needle if it doesn't respond to soaking alone. This isn't an area for partners to be digging into!

The pain usually disappears as soon as the white spot is removed, particularly if any thickened milk is then released. Sadly, however, for some mothers, it will reappear and need repeated treatment

Vasospasm

Sometimes mums feel pain when they are breastfeeding. Despite being natural, sometimes it takes a little time for it to feel natural and easy. As the mum's help and support team, you may be useful in watching what is happening during and after a feed.

If you can see that her nipple has a white area on the tip after a feed, and that it looks flattened or lipstick shaped, it is likely that she needs help from an expert with skills in helping breastfeeding mothers. The white tip to the nipple suggests that the baby is squashing the nipple between gum or tongue and the roof of his mouth. This effectively cuts off the blood supply to the nipple, which is why it goes white. As the blood flows back, it sets off all the nerve endings in this very sensitive area, which is what causes the excruciating pain that goes on for some time. There are no drugs or creams to fix this; just an expert to improve the attachment.

It can be a symptom of tongue-tie when the baby is unable to move the tongue in the right way to extract the milk. It can also occur from around 2 weeks after birth, when the baby notices that the milk is flowing too fast, and uses his tongue to slow the flow down, effectively squeezing the nipple to prevent himself from choking.

Raynaud's Phenomenon

Raynaud's phenomenon is associated with poor circulation. Sufferers will be used to the sight of white fingers and toes, and the need to wrap up warmly in the winter. Raynaud's affects up to 10% of otherwise healthy women, aged 21 to 50 years.

The symptoms of Raynaud's (as they affect breastfeeding) are pain after mothers breastfeed. This happens immediately, as the nipple comes out of the baby's mouth and becomes cooler. The nipples undergo a rapid colour change from white to purple, and then red, as shown below, taken by a mother on her cell phone (Holmen & Backe, 2009). Pain can also come on when the mother is in a cold situation (e.g., passing the freezer section in a super-market). She may automatically cover her nipples as she stops feeding, or rub them between her finger and thumb.

Raynaud's is 9 times more common in women than men. When a mother with Raynaud's is breastfeeding, the poor circulation can extend to the nipples. She is also more likely to deliver her baby early, and for it to be of lower than average birthweight due to restricted blood flow through the placenta. (Arnold et al., 2015; Kahl eet al., 1990).

It is possible that she may not have had symptoms of Raynaud's in the past herself, but has a close family member who does. It can also be linked to severe migraines, and with autoimmune conditions, such as scleroderma, rheumatoid arthritis, Sjogren's syndrome, and lupus. Around 1 in 10 people with Raynaud's go on to develop an autoimmune condition (www.nhs.uk/conditions/raynauds-phenomenon/pages/causes.aspx).

There are some self-help measures that can help to relieve symptoms of Raynaud's.

- ⊙ Stop smoking. Even 2 cigarettes a day is enough to reduce blood flow by 40%.

- ⊙ Limit caffeine intake (both nicotine and caffeine constrict blood vessels). Caffeine is not just in tea and coffee, but also in soft and energy drinks, as well as some painkillers.

- ⊙ Avoid getting cold.

- ⊙ Try gentle aerobic exercise (Cardelli,1989). Rub the nipples gently with warm oil immediately after feeds, or cover the breast immediately with a warm, heat-retaining compress (e.g., wheat bag).

- ⊙ Avoid decongestants (in cold remedies), the combined contraceptive pill, and fluconazole (used to treat thrush), which can make symptoms worse.

Supplements of high doses of vitamin B6 (Kernerman & Newman, 2015), magnesium (Leppert et al., 1994; Smith, Hammarsten, & Eliel, 1960; Turlapaty & Alture, 1980), calcium (DiGiacomo, 1989), fatty acids (Belch et al., 1985), and fish-oil supplementation have been suggested, but take a minimum of 6 weeks to be effective in relieving symptoms. Anecdotally, ginger supplements of 2000 to 4000 mg daily have also been recommended to prevent and relieve symptoms. Capsules usually contain 500 mg. It may also be beneficial to add ginger to the diet, or to drink ginger tea, according to the Scleroderma and Raynaud's UK (https://www.sruk.co.uk/, although there appears no research to support this.

Symptoms can be successfully managed by the use of a drug called nifedipine, 30 mg daily (10 mg capsules, three times a day, or long-acting tablet 30 mg daily) for 2 weeks. This has to be prescribed by a doctor. Some women need to keep taking medication long term, but many find that the symptoms disappear after 2 weeks. However, the drug produces hot flashes and headaches, which some women find difficult to tolerate.

Too Much Milk

It is interesting that some mothers make more milk than their babies can easily cope with. This is quite common in the first few weeks of breastfeeding, but for some mothers, it can continue for longer.

You can help the mum's supply adjust to your baby's needs by making sure your baby's attachment on the breast is as good as it can be. If the mum's breasts are full and uncomfortable, it is fine to wake the baby to feed; demand feeding should work both ways! It may work for the mum to feed more frequently so that her breasts don't get too full, and then the baby ends up choking on the large volume of milk released quickly. It can be useful to express as necessary and store the milk

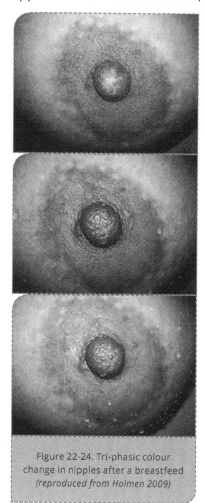

Figure 22-24. Tri-phasic colour change in nipples after a breastfeed (reproduced from Holmen 2009)

for days when you want to go out as a couple, or even to mix with solids later.

If your daughter or partner finds it easy to express this additional milk, it would be a wonderful gesture to donate this to a milk bank (www.ukamb.org). This milk is given to premature and sick babies who cannot receive their own mother's milk. It can save lives, and gets babies home with their parents sooner.

Moving on from Breastfeeding

Weaning from the Breast

When we talk about weaning, we have to differentiate between reducing milk feeds as the baby begins to take more solids, the cessation of breastfeeding, and replacement of breastmilk with other liquids.

According to the 2010 Infant Feeding Survey, there are still 63% of women who stopped breastfeeding before they intended, although 7% managed to feed for longer than they had initially planned.

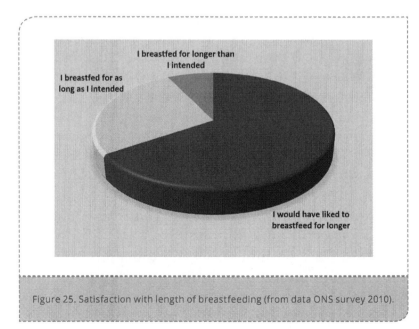

Figure 25. Satisfaction with length of breastfeeding (from data ONS survey 2010).

Age of baby	Proportion of babies breastfed %
Birth	81
2 days	76
3 days	74
4 days	72
5 days	71
6 days	70
1 week	69
2 weeks	66
6 weeks	55
4 months	42
6 months	34
9 months	23

Table 5. Proportion of babies breastfed with increasing age.

Why do Mothers Stop Breastfeeding Sooner than they Intended?

For the most part, in the first 2 weeks, the majority of reasons given could all be explained by the mother and baby not having achieved good attachment, which we have already discussed leads to painful nipples and poor milk supply. If this happens in your new family, you need to phone a friendly breastfeeding expert to help. Nipples should not be painful during a breastfeed. Why would Nature make something you need to do 8 to 12 times a day so painful that you would do anything to avoid it? The vast majority of women (at least 98%) can produce enough milk to satisfy their baby. However, sometimes we cause problems by trying to schedule feeds, keeping the mum and baby apart, or not helping the mum achieve a pain-free latch.

Reasons giving for stopping later on are more complicated, but sadly may still relate to painful feeds or milk production, but phrased in other ways. The right time for weaning from the breast is an individual choice. What makes me sad is when women regret the decision they have made, and may even feel guilty.

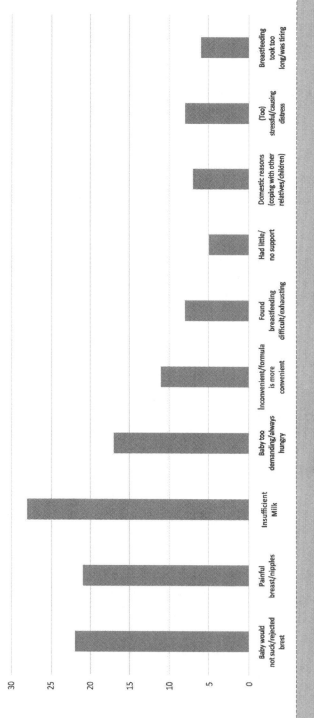

Figure 26. Reasons given for stopping breastfeeding in the first 2 weeks after birth.

So much of the heated debate in the media about pro-breast-feeding and formula-milk feeding seems to be based on anger that they did not receive help when they had problems, or that their concerns were not listened to with appropriate support being offered.

	4 weeks to 4 months	4 to 10 months
	%	%
Baby not feeding properly/enough/not interested	18	18
Baby ill	11	14
Baby vomiting/reflux	10	7
Breast milk dried up/not enough	10	3
Needed (top-ups of) formula milk	9	6
Breastfeeding uncomfortable or painful (including sore breasts/nipples/mastitis)	9	6
Not gaining enough weight/lost weight	8	2
Colic/wind	8	1
Baby still hungry/not satisfied/waking at night	6	3
Baby lactose intolerant	5	3
Wouldn't suck/latch on/poor attachment	5	3
Baby (had to be) started on solids	4	10
Problems related to feeding solids	4	37
Wouldn't take bottle	4	5
Baby teething	3	12
Blocked milk duct	2	1
Had to change formula milk	1	2
Baby prefers breast/only wants formula/cow's milk	0	11

Table 6. Reasons given for stopping breastfeeding up to 10 months

There continues to be benefits in breastfeeding to 2 years of age and beyond. It seems many people are ready to question why mothers continue to breastfeed past a year. Breastmilk still provides nutrition, immunity, and comfort in a challenging world. There is no reason to stop unless you choose to. If we compare ourselves to other mammals and the time at which they naturally wean, it would be around 5 years of age. For more information, look at Dr. Kathy Dettwyler's website http://kathydettwyler.weebly.com/. Kathy is an anthropologist with an interest in birth and breastfeeding.

But if long-term breastfeeding isn't right for you as a family, that's fine too. We are all individuals making our own choices of what is right for us. What upsets me is when people criticise each other. Life is too short to be nasty to each other. Live and let live.

Weaning onto Solids

Current research advises that exclusive breastfeeding—that is, offering nothing except breastmilk and medicine—provides the baby with the best nutrition and long-term protection.

Grandma, when we had our children, the advice was very different. When I had my eldest, it was when the baby weighed 12 lb, or was 3 months old, whichever came first. By the time I had my youngest, 7 years later, it was 4 months. When we were babies, it was not uncommon to add rusk to the bottles of very young babies to help them sleep.

So why the change? Does it matter? Yes, it does matter if we look at the research on the nutritional needs of babies, and the benefit of no other substances being introduced to the gut, which may decrease the protection. It is also recommended that by waiting until 6 months, we no longer need to introduce spoon-fed baby rice or purees, but can offer foods that the baby can hold and eat alone.

A baby shows readiness to wean by being able to:

- Sit up independently and hold their head up steadily.
- Coordinate putting food into the mouth by themselves. This entails developing hand-eye movement.
- The ability to take food to the back of the mouth. If you offer food too soon, most of it is pushed back out.

Milk provides the majority of the baby's nutritional needs to 12 months, which allows him time to taste and explore other tastes. There is no rush to introduce large quantities of food at each meal. Indeed, that will increase the risk of obesity by rapid weight gain.

From around 6 months, your baby's first foods can include soft cooked vegetables like parsnip, potato, sweet potato, or carrot. Soft fresh fruit, like banana or avocado, are often early favourites. They can be offered as finger foods or mashed up. Although you can spoon-feed the baby, you may be surprised how good they are at doing this themselves (worth having a large washable mat underneath the high chair though).

Wanting extra milk feeds and waking at night or chewing fists is not a sign of being ready for solids. These behaviours are common from 4 to 6 months. Rarely are baby's bodies ready for foods other than milk before 6 months regardless of their weight.

You can use cow's milk to cook from 6 months, or breastmilk, so there is no need to buy formula milk (particularly follow-on formula milk, which despite adverts, has no nutritional advantages over breast or normal formula milk). You can also offer sips of water after a meal from a cup so there's no need to introduce bottles.

There is lots of good information in the leaflet produced by the NHS Introducing Solid Foods www.nhs.uk/start4life/documents/pdfs/introducing_solid_foods.pdf.

Each child is an individual and will take to solids at his own pace. This isn't a competition to see who can take 3 meals a day first. It is developing an appreciation to try tastes, and experiment with textures of food, which last our whole lives.

Expressing
Breastmilk

Expressing

The question of expressing in order for Dad to offer a bottle over-night to give mum a chance to sleep is frequently raised. However, well-intentioned as this is, it sadly isn't helpful, particularly in the early weeks.

Remember how we discussed the hormones that affect milk supply in Chapter 4? If the mother expresses milk to put into the bottle, she will need to express at the time the feed is due. If she doesn't, she may risk a blocked duct from milk leaking in the breast (or at the very least, be woken by aching breasts). In addition, if the milk is not removed, then FIL will tell her body that it does not need to make as much milk for the next feed. The result is likely to be an unhappy mum and baby in the morning, and a dad frustrated that he had an interrupted night sleep, and it hasn't really helped! If you want to help your partner get more sleep, then bring her breakfast, and even lunch, in bed. Spend time with your baby when he is awake, and leave the feeding to the mum.

However, there will come a day when you want to go out as a couple, or mum has an appointment, and a bottle of expressed breastmilk is needed. It is useful to learn how to hand express breastmilk, and according to the Baby-Friendly Initiative, this tech-nique should be taught to all mothers. It is useful for the following reasons.

- It can be done anywhere, anytime. No need to have a pump available.
- It can be used to relieve symptoms of blocked duct or mastitis.

- ⊙ It can relieve engorgement so that the breast is softened and easier to latch onto.

- ⊙ If the mother and baby are separated, e.g., if baby is preterm, the mother can provide her milk.

- ⊙ If the baby is sleepy in the first few days after delivery, expressing a little and dribbling it into his mouth may tempt him to wake up and feed. If necessary, the colostrum can be dribbled into the baby's mouth by a small medicine syringe or spoon.

- ⊙ Expressing milk can convince you all that there really is milk there.

- ⊙ It will help you understand how far back from the nipple the breast produces milk (you can feel the change in tissue if you explore it very gently), and that will show you why a deep latch is needed.

- ⊙ Some mothers do not like the feeling of using pumps, be they manual or electric.

- ⊙ You can use expressed milk as eye drops for eye infections!

A video showing you how to hand express is available here: www.unicef.org.uk/BabyFriendly/Resources/AudioVideo/Hand-expression/.

Further written information and in a video can be found here: www.nhs.uk/conditions/pregnancy-and-baby/pages/expressing-storing-breast-milk.aspx#close.

However, not everyone can master the art of hand expressing. My daughter, who gave birth to a slightly premature baby, couldn't bear watching the colostrum appear on her nipples. She desperately wanted to provide the vital nourishment, but had to leave it to others to hand express and collect it. That was apparently my role!

There are a variety of hand-operated and electric breast pumps. The choice is purely personal, and no one is superior to all the others. You may be guided by friends and colleagues who have used them. Hand or electric depends on how often you are going to use one. Are you returning to work, or expressing for comfort and occasional bottles left while you are out? My eldest daughter had to go back to work full-time when her son was 4 months old. She needed an electric double-pump for efficiency and to save time.

Returning to Work

Some mothers have to return to work while breastfeeding. It is possible to express milk to leave for the baby to have during her absence. It can feel daunting, and to some people, very unnatural. If there is childcare available that is close to her workplace, she may be able to visit your baby during the lunch hour to breastfeed. Employers should provide somewhere for the mother to express in privacy and a fridge to store the milk.

A large employer may have a special "mother and baby room." In other workplaces, you may be able to use a first-aid room, spare office, or a private room, preferably with a lockable door so that she can relax.

How often you should express milk is very individual. It depends on the age of the baby, and how much milk is needed during the mum's absence. Just as with breastfeeding, the more frequently the mum expresses, the greater volume she will make. Some people find the whole process stressful, and it is important to try to relax to allow the oxytocin to release the milk. It may be that the mum can use an electric breast pump with dual breast collection. These can be used in a special "bra," which holds them in place, allowing the mum access to her mobile phone, tablet, or computer so that she can "work" at the same time. Or she can take the opportunity to nap or read a book. Technology makes most options possible.

In an ideal world, the mum would be able to take expressing breaks whenever she needs to. This may be a time when the baby would normally feed or she feels full. However, realistically, this may need to fit in with work demands. So long as she is not uncomfortable, it doesn't really matter, so long as she can fit in enough expressing sessions to produce the milk needed by the baby the following day.

For information on breastfeeding and returning to work there is an excellent leaflet by Maternity Action: www.maternityaction. org.uk/sitebuildercontent/sitebuilderfiles/breastfeeding.pdf.

For more information on expression and storage of breastmilk, see: www.breastfeedingnetwork.org.uk/wp-content/pdfs/ BFNExpressing_and_Storing.pdf.

Employers may need reminding that breastfed babies have fewer illness and recover faster than artificially fed infants, and that long term this will mean that the mother will have to take less time off to care for her child. So provision of facilities to help breastfeeding is a good investment. It is also true that employers who look after the needs of their staff have lower staff turnover, which is a further economic advantage. If there are queries that you have, it is better to ask the Human Resource Department, who should have greater knowledge of the law and work practices than line-managers.

It is a good idea to keep bottles of expressed breastmilk in small volumes to avoid waste. Once a baby has started to suck on a bottle of milk, anything left after an hour has to be thrown away, as the risk of stomach bugs increases dramatically after this time. There is nothing worse than throwing away 4 oz (120 ml) from a 5 oz bottle as the baby wasn't that hungry. All that effort! This is one time when you do cry over spilled milk.

When the mum returns to work, you may find that the little one doesn't drink as much during the day when away from the mum, but feeds avidly when he is back with her. This is called reverse-cy-cling. Sometimes it is reassuring for the mother to re-establish the pre-work relationship and bonding. But let's be honest; it can be tiring too. Sorry, Dad, you may be needed to help cook or bathe the baby, and generally be supportive.

Getting the baby to take a bottle is often discussed on social media as a nightmare for mothers preparing to go back to work. Which bottle? Which nipple? What if he won't drink from a bottle? Or he used to take a bottle, but won't now?

There is no reason why a baby older than 6 months needs to take his milk from a bottle; a sippy cup will do. Other children will drink really well from a simple cup. I was taught, 35 years ago, to use a fine china cup.

It is not unusual for a baby to refuse a bottle from his mother. Why should he when he knows the "tap" is nearby? He may take the bottle from you or Grandma. Even if he takes very little when in daycare, it is likely that he will make up for it overnight. Watch out for dry nappies as a sign of dehydration. Breastmilk should be stored in the fridge, or in a cool bag with ice packs, if possible. It is a living fluid, but can still become contaminated if not handled with care.

If You Decide to Formula-Feed Your Baby

I have spoken to several fathers and grandmothers who have been concerned about switching to formula-feeding the baby at whatever the age. It may be that you need to give just a few bottles: when everything gets to be too much, if the mum is ill, if the mum has to take medication that isn't compatible with breastfeeding (rare: Please email me before you make that decision), or has to be away from the baby. It may also be that you, as a family, have decided that this is the right time to stop breastfeeding the baby.

What Milk Does to a Non-Breastfed Baby?

Formula milk is needed to nourish a baby under 12 months of age if he is not being breastfed. Beyond one year, there is no need to use formula milk, but the baby can move straight onto full-fat cow's milk. There is no benefit in using Follow-On formula milk, rather than simple whey- or casein-dominant milk. It was developed to bypass the advertising regulations on breastmilk substitutes.

What Bottle is Best?

Beyond 6 months, babies do not need to take bottles, but can take milk from a cup, if they prefer. Stirling, at 9 months, refused point-blank to take his expressed milk at the nursery from a bottle any longer, despite having done so during the day from 3 months. He preferred a cup with a straw. Every baby is different. Some enjoy the feel/taste/texture of any teat, while others are very fussy. Cups come with straws built into the lid, with soft spouts, or with normal spouts. It is possible to use a normal cup without a lid, a Doidy cup, which is shaped with a slant for easy drinking, an egg cup, or a plastic beaker. In the transition, you may have to be flexible until you find out what works for you and your baby.

How to Make Up a Bottle of Formula Milk

Ready-prepared formula milk sold in cartons is sterile and can be used as it is. Powered formula milk is not sterile, so it should be made fresh for each feed.

Hygiene

Before preparing the formula milk, wash your hands and the surface on which you will prepare the bottle well with hot, soapy water. The bottle should have been washed, rinsed, and sterilised. Dishwashers will wash bottles, but do not reach high enough temperatures to sterilise them. Milk is an ideal medium on which bacteria can grow and multiply, so hygiene standards must be followed carefully if you are to avoid your baby getting gastroenteritis.

Bottles and nipples can be sterilised in a variety of means:

- Using a cold-water sterilising solution,
- Steam sterilising, or
- Sterilising by boiling.

To reduce the risk of infection, each feed should be made up as your baby needs it, using freshly boiled tap water at a temperature of at least 70°C. Do not use water that has been previously boiled, as this concentrates any impurities (e.g., calcium carbonate in a hard-water area). Do not use artificially softened water or bottled water to make up formula milk. The latter contains a variable amount of salt and/or sulphate. If use is necessary because of the risk of contaminated tap water, it still needs to be heated to 70°C.

Water at 70°C will kill any harmful bacteria that may be present in the powdered formula milk. The formula milk should then be allowed to cool before being given to the baby. This may be hastened by running the bottle under a running cold water tap (avoiding the nipple). Previously boiled water that has cooled below 70°C cannot kill all the potentially harmful organisms.

what you need for formula feeding

You need to make sure you clean and sterilise the equipment to prevent your baby from getting infections and stomach upsets. You'll need:

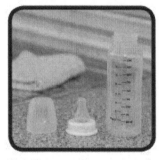

bottles with teats and bottle covers

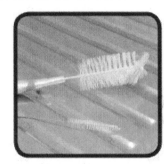

bottle brush, teat brush

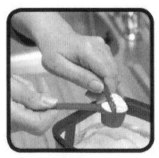

formula milk powder, or sterile ready-to-feed liquid formula

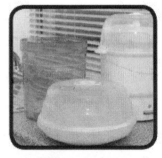

sterilising equipment (such as a cold-water steriliser, microwave or steam steriliser)

Figure 27. What you need to formula feed
www.unicef.org.uk/Documents/Baby_Friendly/Leaflets/guide_to_bottle_feeding.pdf

cold-water sterilising solution

- Follow the manufacturer's instructions.
- Change the sterilising solution every 24 hours.
- Leave feeding equipment in the sterilising solution for at least 30 minutes.
- Make sure that there is no air trapped in the bottles or teats when putting them in the sterilising solution.
- Keep all the equipment under the solution with a floating cover.

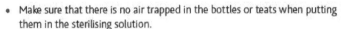

steam sterilising (electric steriliser or microwave)

- As there are different types of steriliser it is important to follow the manufacturer's instructions.
- Make sure the openings of the bottles and teats are facing down in the steriliser.
- Manufacturers will give a guide as to how long you can leave equipment that you are not using straight after sterilising before it needs to be resterilised.

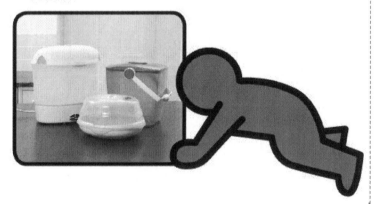

Figure 28. Sterilisation of bottles
www.unicef.org.uk/Documents/Baby_Friendly/Leaflets/guide_to_bottle_feeding.pdf

Making Up a Bottle of Formula Milk

Ensure that you are using a scoop provided by the manufacturer of the brand you are using, as they vary slightly in volume. It does not matter which brand you use, as they all have to contain the ingredients proven to be necessary to the health and development of the baby.

1. Fill the kettle with sufficient freshly drawn tap water and bring it to the boil. It may be left to cool in the kettle, but for no longer than 30 minutes, or the temperature may have fallen below the required 70°C.

2. Before touching the bottles, nipples, or powdered formula milk, wash your hands thoroughly.

3. Rinse any excess sterilising fluid from the bottle using the boiled water from the kettle. Ensure that you don't leave the nipple on an unsterilised surface while you make up the bottle.

4. Pour the volume of hot water required for the volume of feed into the bottle from the kettle.

5. Loosely fill the scoop with formula milk according to the manufacturer's instructions, and level it off using either the flat edge of a clean, dry knife or the leveller provided. Adding too much formula milk powder will over-concentrate the feed and can lead to constipation, dehydration, and illness. This can happen easily by adding heaped scoops, or pressing the powder down into the scoop. Adding too little formula milk powder can lead to lack of nutrition and poor weight gain.

6. Put the teat onto the bottle, taking care not to handle the part which will go into the baby's mouth, and replace the ring holding it in place. Cover with the lid.

7. Shake the bottle thoroughly so that all the formula milk powder is dissolved in the water.

8. Cool the bottle under cold running water until the formula milk, if dropped onto the inside of your wrist, is a comfortable temperature.

9. Offer the bottle to the baby.

If you are using cartons of ready-to-feed formula milk, you can pour the contents straight into the sterilised bottle and add the teat. Some babies prefer the milk warmed in a jug of hot water, while others are happy to drink it as room temperature. Formula milk should never be heated in a microwave, as it is easy for it to overheat or heat unevenly, which could result in scalding the baby's mouth.

Feeding the Baby

Feed your baby when he shows signs of being hungry, just as you did when he was being breastfed. Watch for the same cues (moving head and mouth around, sucking on fingers), rather than watching the clock.

Crying is the last sign of wanting to feed, so try and feed your baby before he cries. This is especially true with formula-feeding when you consider how long it will take you to prepare the bottle compared with breastfeeding. Crying with hunger is frustrating for the baby, who will swallow more air, and frustrating for you as you try to keep the baby settled, especially during night feeds.

Your baby will know how much milk he needs. The amount needed per feed, according to the manufacturer's instructions on the tin, is a guide only, and there is no need to force your baby to finish the bottle. This can be distressing to the baby (imagine being forced to clear every forkful of food from your plate, regardless of how full you feel), and can lead to overfeeding and excessive weight gain. You will soon recognise your baby's cues that he has had enough milk.

Before you begin, make sure that you are comfortable and relaxed. Hold your baby close in a semi-upright position, so you can see his face and reassure him by looking into his eyes and talking to him during the feed. Remember that we discussed the importance of the baby's position when breastfeeding with the head and body needing to be in a straight line, with no twisting of the neck, or neck forced downwards onto the chest. Babies who are just transitioning onto formula-feeding may feel more comfortable being held in skin to skin for a while.

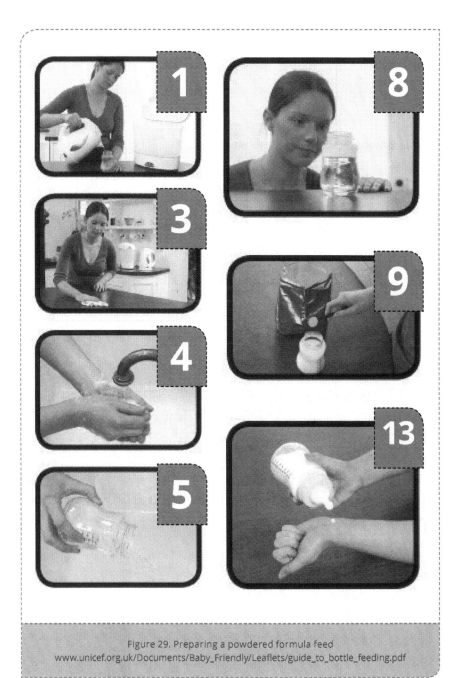

Figure 29. Preparing a powdered formula feed
www.unicef.org.uk/Documents/Baby_Friendly/Leaflets/guide_to_bottle_feeding.pdf

Gently rub the nipple along the baby's top lip to encourage him to open his mouth wide and take the nipple into his mouth. Do not force the nipple into the baby's mouth. Hold the nipple just higher than the horizontal so that the nipple is kept full of milk at all times.

After the feed, or for some babies during the feed, the baby may need to burp. To do this, sit the baby up on your lap, or over your shoulder, and gently rub his back.

Storing Formula Feeds

A feed should be freshly made up when it is needed to reduce the risk of sickness and diarrhoea. Any infant formula milk left in the bottle after a feed should be thrown away within an hour. Infant formula milk that has been made up, but not been used, and has been kept at room temperature, must be thrown away within 2 hours. Even if a feed is kept in a fridge, bacteria can still survive and multiply, although they do this more slowly than at room temperature.

The risk of infection increases over time, so that is why it is important to make up the feed each time your baby needs it. Once opened, any unused liquid infant formula milk that remains in the carton needs to be stored at the back of the fridge, on the top shelf, with the cut corner turned down, and for no longer than 24 hours.

Remember, bottle-feeding formula milk can and should be safe and responsive feeding.

More Information

For more information, please check these resources:

- ⊙ **First Steps Nutrition Infant Milks in the UK**
  www.firststepsnutrition.org/pdfs/Infant_Milks_June_2015.pdf

- ⊙ **Unicef UK Baby-Friendly Initiative**
  A guide to infant formula for parents who are bottle-feeding which can be downloaded at www.unicef.org.uk/Documents/Baby_Friendly/Leaflets/guide_infant_formula.pdf

⊙ **Start4Life Guide to Bottle-Feeding**

www.gov.uk/government/uploads/system/uploads/
attachment_data/file/212827/2900017-Bottle-feeding-leaflet-
v1_0-no-crops.pdf

When a Breastfeeding Mother May Need to Take Medicine

The safety of drugs in breastmilk is my area of expertise, and the topic of my first book, *Breastfeeding and Medication*, so it doesn't feel right to miss out on a section on common illnesses, and which medications can be taken by a mother who is breastfeeding. You and she may be worried that she can't take anything.

We avoid as many drugs as possible in pregnancy, so does this apply to breastfeeding? Can we contaminate breastmilk to the point where formula milk would be better? In a tiny number of cases, this is true. In most cases, she can take medication, and continue to breastfeed as normal.

The leaflet in most medicine boxes says not to take it if you are breastfeeding, or to consult your GP or pharmacist before doing so. This does not indicate risk, just that the manufacturers are not required to take responsibility for use in breastfeeding mothers because clinical studies are unethical. This information does not have to change, no matter how long the product is available or how much we know about the safety of the product in breastmilk.

What to Do if Your Partner/Daughter is Told to Stop Breastfeeding in Order to Take a Medication

As I have already told you, my special role for the last 30 years has been to support mothers who have been prescribed, or purchased a medicine to continue to breastfeed. Although this book is not about this topic, and I have already published that under the title

Breastfeeding and Medication, I cannot let the opportunity pass to remind you, as a supporter of breastfeeding, that if the most important woman in our life is told to stop breastfeeding under these circumstances, that you need to seek help. I can be contacted via my website www.breastfeeding-and-medication.co.uk, or my Facebook page, Breastfeeding and Medication. Do not assume that there is no alternative that allows breastfeeding to continue. I will gladly provide you with the research so that you can make your own informed decisions.

Conditions Affecting Mental Health

Anxiety

Many mothers (and fathers and grandmothers) are anxious after the arrival of the baby. It is totally natural, as we are in very unfamiliar territory where we want to do everything perfectly. It doesn't matter if this isn't your first baby. You haven't met this little person before, and he may not have the same needs or routines as other babies. You may have younger brothers and sisters, but you have not had to take ultimate 24-hour-a-day responsibility for a baby in the same way.

Anxiety is really common in new mothers–more common than depression. Having a baby is an exciting time, full of intense emotions, but too much anxiety can interfere with ability to cope with daily activities and enjoying life. Depression, anxiety, and panic attacks are not signs of weakness. They are signs of having tried to remain strong for too long

With a new baby, you may be having problems with sleep deprivation, too many visitors, and no time to eat (let alone prepare a hot meal). Mum may have sore nipples or pain when she poos because of the bruising of stitches (sorry if that is too much information). You may all be worried that the baby is not putting on enough weight, is sleeping too much or not enough, and you may be confused about the best place to put the baby to sleep, conflicting advice, and information in books that all differs from each other. All of these factors can cause anxiety.

In one study, 17% of mothers described themselves as anxious at 2 weeks, while 6% were depressed (Paul et al., 2013). It is common and many mothers experience it. Anxiety can be totally debilitating, and you may need some help if it isn't reducing. You are not going mad. The symptoms of anxiety are listed below.

Symptoms of anxiety
⊙ Trouble concentrating and remembering things
⊙ Difficulties finishing everyday tasks
⊙ Trouble making decisions
⊙ Difficulty relaxing
⊙ Insomnia
⊙ Exhaustion
⊙ Feelings of extreme uneasiness for prolonged periods of time
⊙ Loss of appetite
⊙ Possible suicidal thoughts
⊙ Anxiety/panic attacks

Table 7. Symptoms of anxiety

Signs of a panic attack
⊙ Shortness of breath
⊙ Feeling of being choked or smothered
⊙ Chest pain or discomfort
⊙ Heart palpitations or increased heart rate
⊙ Hot flushes or chills
⊙ Sweating
⊙ Trembling or shaking
⊙ Tingling sensation
⊙ Feeling faint, dizzy, lightheaded, or unsteady
⊙ Nausea or stomach upset
⊙ Depersonalization (feeling removed or disoriented from the world)
⊙ Fear of going mad or doing something uncontrolled
⊙ Sense of impending doom or death

Table 8. Signs of a panic attack

If you, Dad or Grandma, hear the mum saying:

⊙ "My thoughts are racing." This may be a sign of a more serious condition, so may need urgent medical help.

⊙ "I can't focus on anything."

⊙ "I find it hard to make decisions."

⊙ "I can't relax."

Then she is probably suffering from anxiety and/or depression, and needs some help. When we are anxious, our bodies produce lots of adrenaline, which works against oxytocin. This means that the baby can be unsettled, as the let-down may take longer. This further intensifies anxiety around not having enough milk and being able to satisfy the baby. One mother emailed me with this comment.

> Whilst I've always struggled with anxiety, it spilled over and came to a peak last night, resulting in a break-down. As a results, my milk supply is extremely low, and the worse is that I don't seem to be having a let-down anymore (last was 7 pm last night).

After a supportive discussion about the effect of adrenaline on oxytocin, she sent the following message.

> You were absolutely right! I had a friend over this after-noon and have been able to feed twice since.

However, it is important that the mum also discusses how she feels with her medical team. In an ideal world, access to "Talking Therapies," such as Cognitive-Behavioural Therapy (CBT) would be the best option, allowing her to explore why she feels anxious, and how she can control it herself. In reality, access is not so easy. For example, current government in the UK-promised targets are that all people with any mental health symptoms (don't worry, I say again she isn't going mad) will get access within 13 weeks. Mothers with young babies should be prioritised, but in many cases, will be expected to attend without their baby in order to gain maximum benefit from the sessions. If you think about it, it is often hard to finish a sentence with a new baby in your arms. To challenge thought pattern in these circumstances would be impossible. Dad or Grandma, can you help by looking after the baby or helping, maybe, to pay for childcare?

So the option is to consider some medication, alongside reducing caffeine intake and taking some exercise. A brisk walk is fine. The option I would choose first is a beta blocker, such as propranolol (Inderal ®). This drug has been used for anxiety and panic for many years, and is very effective. It is not appropriate if the mum has asthma. In addition, it passes into breastmilk in such small quantities that it should not affect the breastfed baby.

Some mothers need to take it regularly, 3 times a day until the symptoms diminish, while others can take it when needed.

Alongside the beta blocker, your GP may consider an antidepressant, not because anxiety is depression (although it may be incorrectly diagnosed as such), but because all antidepressants have anti-anxiety effects. The drug of choice would be sertraline (Lustral®, Zoloft®), which should be taken in the morning. This also passes into breastmilk in small levels, and does not affect babies.

Just acknowledging that she feels anxious can help the mother, and if she discusses it with other mums, I will guarantee most of them will be able to identify with her. Do not be afraid of the idea of admitting to a mental health issue. Mental health is just the same as physical health. Sometimes we are running on empty, and sometimes we have a full tank. It is common in the immediate postnatal period, as there are so many demands on new parents to "get it right." As a Grandma, maybe you can reassure the parents that "good enough" is just fine.

One study looked at a group of 28 women with babies between birth and 18 months of age (Conrad & Adams, 2012). The women were divided into two groups, with similar levels of anxiety and depression at the beginning of the study. Those in the study group were given a 15-minute aromatherapy massage twice a week for 4 weeks using Rose otto and lavender essential oils. At 2 and 4 weeks, those receiving the massages had less anxiety and depression with no adverse effects. Could you, Dad or Grandma, give the mum a gentle, encouraging, and relaxing massage to show how much you love her? It need only be a neck message to help calm her down, and could be with any moisturising lotion or oil. We all respond to a loving touch by releasing oxytocin, which reduces adrenaline, the hormone linked with stress.

Depression

> *"What do you mean you are depressed? Why would you be low when you have a lovely new baby? Pull yourself together!"*

That is the sort of comment that some people, sadly, make to new mothers. It isn't helpful, and it further demotivates them, and

133

adds to their feelings of confusion because they may be thinking the same thing.

Partners and mothers may be the first to notice that a new mother is just not quite herself. Most common symptoms begin in the first 4 to 6 weeks after having the baby. In some cases, it may not develop for several months. However, there is increasing evidence that depression may start antenatally.

It is common to feel mood swings and tearfulness in the first few days after birth. If you, as supporters of the mother, are telling her she is doing well, she may burst into tears. If she feels she can't settle the baby as well as you, she may burst into tears. A sad story on the news may have the same result. This is all normal and due to the upheaval in hormones after delivery. She just needs lots of hugs.

As a loving partner, make time to care for the new mum: bring her a cup of tea, maybe a treat she particularly likes, but above all, make sure she knows that you love her just as she is. As a new grandma, maybe you can remember feeling this way yourself. Look after your daughter, and help her to care for her baby. Reassure her that she is a wonderful mother, and how much her baby (and you) love her.

Sometimes symptoms go on for longer, and may intensify. Your partner/daughter may put everything down to being tired, and may deny anything is wrong. Many of us women believe we are "Superwoman"—able to deal with a baby 24 hours a day, carry on with the housework and cooking as normal, play with the baby, and be a good partner, all with less than 4 hours of sleep (on a good day) in one go.

Symptoms of postnatal depression vary from one person to another. They include low mood, increasing inability to cope, difficulty sleeping or being tired all the time, not wanting to go out, eating more or less than usual, getting easily angered, or being tearful. Many symptoms of depression are non-specific (e.g., tiredness, where she wakes up, but yearns to go back to sleep, or doesn't want to get up). She may have an increasing inability to cope as the day goes on. Or she wants to go to bed early. She may lose confidence, and or have an increasing desire to withdraw and avoid socialisation.

There are a wide range of reasons for why mothers get depressed. It seems to be increasingly treated, but is that because we recognise it more now? It can be very frightening, and make the new mother feel that she is a failure. It isn't possible, or sensible, to ignore the symptoms. It is an illness and needs help and support, as well as gentle understanding, just as if she had a physical illness

It is all too easy to dismiss concerns, and not admit that life is not a bed of roses. Mum may be scared that if she admits she feels very low and is having difficulty coping, that Social Services may become involved, and in the worst case scenario, they will remove her baby from her care.

This truly is not going to happen! Everyone wants to help and support you as a new family. Dad and Grandma, you may feel depressed too, as being alongside someone who is low reflects in your own feelings. Depression has been called "The Black Dog," and the "Thief who Steals Motherhood."

In 2006, it was reported that breastfeeding mothers have lower rates of depression than artificially feeding mothers (Groer & Davis, 2006). Researchers identified that the mothers who are not exclusively breastfeeding have a more hyperactive stress and inflammation response, which puts them at higher risk for depression. Exclusive breastfeeding helps lessen this stress response, and by doing so, decreases the breastfeeding mothers' risk of depression (Kendall-Tackett, 2007). This is true even for mothers who have experienced significant psychological trauma, including sexual assault (Kendall-Tackett, Cong, & Hale, 2013).

In 2014, over 10,000 mothers were studied. It was found that women who breastfed their babies were at a significantly lower risk of postnatal depression than those who did not (Borra et al., 2015). The highest risk of depression was found among women who had planned to breastfeed, but were not able to—those who perceived themselves as "failing." For previously depressed mothers, there may also be a protective effect from breastfeeding when mothers had not planned to breastfeed, but did so exclusively for 4 weeks.

135

In general, approximately 15% to 25% of women experience post-natal depression within the 14 weeks after giving birth.

This makes it important that, as a society (and particularly, the most important people in a new mother's life, the father and grandmother of her baby), we should support and encourage new mothers, but never pressure women who feel uncomfortable with breastfeeding for their own reasons. Virtually all mothers can breastfeed, provided that they have accurate information and support from their families, communities, and the health care system. Breastfeeding is natural, but it does not always happen naturally and without problems. Mothers may need active support from their caregivers to establish breastfeeding. They may need you to ask for that help for them. Over the years, I have breastfed myself, and supported other mums, I have never ceased to be amazed at how wonderful nature is in providing such a perfect product for free, on tap all the time, and perfectly packaged.

Risk factors for depression include:

- Previous history of depression
- Family history of depression
- History of psychological trauma
- Painful breastfeeding/breastfeeding problems
- Not "succeeding" at breastfeeding
- Social isolation
- Lack of social support
- Sleep problems
- Traumatic birth experience

If your partner has one or more of these risk factors, it doesn't mean she will inevitably become depressed. It's just that we should be alert for symptoms and treat it sooner rather than later. Anecdotally, some mothers choose to take antidepressants after birth "just in case." For mothers who are at higher risk, it would seem good practice to make sure that she has contact with a breastfeeding expert friend, or even a positive social media group, before the birth. Dad, you are in charge of reminding her to "phone a friend."

There are medicines that can be prescribed for the mum, even if she is breastfeeding. Depression is not a reason to stop breastfeeding and may, in fact, make the symptoms worse because she doesn't get the stress-reducing effects of having the baby at the breast.

So, we are looking at a depressed mother taking antidepressants. There are two different types of antidepressants: tricyclic antidepressants, which have been used for many years. They have side effects that are not ideal for a new mother: drowsiness, constipation, urinary retention, and postural hypotension (get dizzy when you stand up suddenly), but we know a lot about their safety in the breastfeeding mother. Examples are amitriptyline (Tryptizol®, Enovil®), imipramine (Tofranil®), and lofepramine. The only one that is not suitable to be used by a breastfeeding mother is dothiepin (Prothiaden®).

The other type, and more widely prescribed, are the Selective Serotonin Re-uptake Inhibitors (SSRI) family of drugs, that include fluoxetine (Prozac®), Sertraline (Lustral®, Zoloft®), Citalopram (Cipramil®, Celexa®), Escitalopram (Cipralex® Lexapro®), and Paroxetine (Seroxat® Paxil®). These drugs have different side effects, and can make the person taking them feel initially worse by producing headaches and nausea. This normally passes in a few days, and they take up to 4 weeks to reach full effectiveness.

I am frequently asked which drug is the best. The answer is whichever a mother has taken in the past would be first choice, assuming it was effective. For anyone who has never taken an antidepressant, sertraline passes into breastmilk in the lowest levels, and is associated with fewer side effects in the baby due to the low amount passing through breastmilk. The drug that is best avoided in the first 6 weeks after birth is fluoxetine. It is widely used in pregnancy as having the best outcomes. However, for some babies the first few days after birth are a time of concern to everyone. Some, but not all, babies born to mothers taking fluoxetine are very sleepy, and have been described as comatose. This is partly due to the accumulation of drug passed through the placenta, and partly due to the long half-life so that the amount passing through breastmilk can accumulate. The mother may need help to hand express to get as much milk into the baby as possible via syringe or spoon, as necessary.

Long-term, the babies seem to recover and develop normally. Short-term, many are subjected to blood glucose testing and concerns as to whether they need top-ups of formula milk. Unless it has been used and been beneficial previously, it isn't an ideal choice to start in the first 6 weeks as more accumulates in breast-milk than other antidepressants because of the long half-life. Babies with immature kidneys and livers cannot metabolise it as well as older babies do. But if the mum has taken it in the past and finds it effective, it remains a good choice, and breastfeeding can continue as normal. Some babies seem to become sleepy if the mum is taking it, while others become more awake, but whether this is attributable to the drug or a coincidence is debatable,

The benefits of CBT therapy are important in depression too. Morrell and colleagues (2009) gave 89 health visitors additional training to identify depressive symptoms in mothers at 6 to 8 weeks using the Edinburgh Postnatal Depression Score (EPDS), to clinically assess and provide psychologically informed sessions based on CBT or person-centred principles for an hour a week, for 8 weeks. In the control group, mothers were provided usual care. At 6 months, 12.4% in the intervention group had depression compared with 16.7% in the control group. The benefits for the intervention group were maintained at 12 months. This sounds like a wonderful and simple intervention, but we currently have Health Visitors with huge time restraints on basic duties, let alone being able to provide CBT to mothers for an hour a week. As for anxiety, referral for CBT should be a priority. If services are not available, another option is a self-help book. *Feeling Good: The New Mood Therapy* by Dr. David Burns remains a classic for do-it-yourself CBT.

Obsessive Compulsive Disorder (OCD)

OCD is a complex disorder that may surface after birth for the first time, or may have been present before. It is a pattern of behaviours characterised by intrusive thoughts that dominate thinking. For a new mother, it may revolve around the safety of the baby, including a fear that she may harm the baby by accident, or on purpose, or fear germs and infection, or any other significant potential harm. Fear of germs, for example, may be accompanied by compulsive and repetitive cleaning. This is a condition that needs help from an expert. There are many suitable medications to help, and psychological therapies, including CBT, which may help to restore perspective of risk.

Bipolar Disorder

Bipolar disorder, formerly known as manic depression, is a condition that affects moods, which can swing from one extreme to another: depression, where the sufferer feels very low and lethargic, and mania, where they feel very high and may be overactive. This is a complex condition that really requires medication. It can happen for the first time in the postnatal period, and may, at first, look like depression. It is important to seek help right away for bipolar disorder because it can be a cause of postnatal psychosis, and needs to be treated promptly.

It is important that mothers with bipolar disorder do not stop taking medication in order to breastfeed. There are usually options that can manage symptoms and make breastfeeding possible. Drugs include quetiapine (Seroquel®), risperidone (Risperdal®), and olanzapine (Zyprexa®). One drug that is generally not recommended during breastfeeding is lithium (Camcolit®). If bipolar disorder affects your partner, please contact me during pregnancy to discuss the research around the medication that she is on so that you, as a family, can reach an informed decision in conjunction with the health care professionals caring for her.

Post-Traumatic Stress Disorder (PTSD)

PTSD can occur because of a prior trauma, such as previous sexual assault, or after a traumatic delivery (e.g., emergency caesarean section, forceps-delivery, postnatal haemorrhage, or a baby who is seriously ill or premature). Often, in emergency circumstances, midwives and doctors may have to react quickly, and do not have time to explain in detail what is going on, let alone provide choices. Birth trauma can also be caused by harmful or uncaring actions of health care providers. Witnesses to traumatic births, such as dads or grandmas, can also develop PTSD.

If Mum has experienced a traumatic birth, you or the mother may have flashbacks or nightmares of the birth that may leave you in a state of high anxiety. Alternatively, she may have negative thoughts about the birth, and avoid discussing it with her peers or family. In the extreme situation, it may lead to a decision not to have further children. If these thoughts become extreme and do not diminish, it may be possible to meet with a midwife at the hospital where you delivered to discuss what happened and why. It may be that the symptoms appear as anxiety or depression if your caregivers are not listening to your description. Psychological therapy, and an opportunity to debrief and put the experience into perspective, may be useful rather than medication. See the website for Prevention and Treatment of Traumatic Childbirth (PATTCh), for more information on resources available to help overcome a traumatic birth experience (PATTCh.org).

Common Situations Where Medication is Needed

Pain Medications

We all need to take pain medications sometimes. A new mother may need them to deal with the pain of stitches, post-caesarean section, etc. Pain medications basically fall into four different categories:

- Paracetamol
- Aspirin
- Non-steroidal anti-inflammatories, such as ibuprofen
- Opiate painkillers

Paracetamol (Tylenol®) is completely safe to take during breastfeeding at the normal dose of two 500 mg tablets four times a day. Avoid taking Paracetamol in two or more different forms (e.g., in combination with codeine), or together with combination cough and cold remedies. If an older baby needs to be given its own Paracetamol suspension, the breastfeeding mother can continue to take her full dose without worrying about overdosing the baby.

Aspirin should be avoided by breastfeeding mothers. In the 1980s, there were cases of Reye's syndrome. This is a rare syndrome, characterized by acute encephalopathy and fatty degeneration of the liver, usually after a viral illness or chickenpox. The incidence is falling, but sporadic cases are still reported. It was often associated with the use of aspirin during the prodromal illness (before symptoms are obvious). Few cases occur in White children under one year, although it is more common in Black infants in this age group. Many children examined retrospectively show an underlying inborn error of metabolism.

In the absence of an association with Reye's syndrome, aspirin would be a very safe drug to be taken during breastfeeding, as very little passes into breastmilk. If taken accidently, there is no need to panic and dump breastmilk. But do not repeat it. There are no cases of Reye's syndrome associated with the passage of aspirin through breastmilk. Brand names include Dispirin® and Anadin®.

Non-steroidal anti-inflammatory drugs (NSAIDs) include ibuprofen (Nurofen®, Advil®, Motrin®), diclofenac (Voltarol®, Diclomax®, Motifene®, Voltaren®), and naproxen (Naprosyn®, Synflex®). These pass into breastmilk in very small levels, and are safe for breastfeeding mothers. They should be taken with or after food, as they can irritate the stomach lining. If they cause indigestion, they can be taken with a proton pump inhibitor (PPI), such as lansoprazole (Zoton®, Prevacid®) or omeprazole (Losec®, Prilosec®), which protect the stomach and pass into breastmilk in very low levels.

There is less information on the transfer of the newer Cox 2 anti-inflammatories, which are used for patients who are at-risk from gastric bleeding (e.g., celecoxib [Celebrex®]). However, it appears that the amount of celecoxib passing through breastmilk is too small to be harmful.

Opiate drugs include codeine, morphine, and oxycodone. These are much stronger pain medications that are used where Paracetamol or non-steroidal drugs alone, or in combination, have not relieved the pain. Everyone varies in the way they metabolise these drugs in their body. Some metabolise it quickly and concentrate it in their milk, resulting in their baby becoming drowsy, and possibly having difficulty breathing.

Cautious recommendation of use during breastfeeding followed an adverse event report from Canada, where a breastfed baby died at 12 days of age. At post-mortem, he was found to have very high levels of morphine in his blood because his mother had multiple copies of the gene which change codeine into morphine, and was taking high-dose co-codamol for episiotomy pain. The mother had reported side effects of constipation and sleepiness in herself. She had sought medical help on several occasions prior to the baby's death, as he was lethargic and had intermittent periods of difficulty in breastfeeding (Koren et al., 2006).

In another study, it was found that ultra-rapid metabolisers chose to take less codeine than their counterparts complaining of dizziness and constipation (Vander Vaart et al., 2011). They chose instead to take Paracetamol and naproxen, or naproxen alone, which were options in the study protocol.

The MHRA (the Government agency monitoring drug adverse effects) have reported that to date, at least 44 cases of neonatal respiratory depression in breastfed infants of codeine-using mothers have been published (MHRA Codeine, 2015).

Codeine is a drug we want breastfeeding mothers to avoid, if possible. However, there are times when it may be necessary to use it. Observe the baby for sedation, and if it becomes drowsy, stop taking the drug at once. Branded products include Paracetamol #3, #4, Solpadeine®, Ultramol®, and Paracodol®. Codeine is also a constituent of a wide variety of preparations available over the counter, which contain multiple analgesic ingredients (e.g., Veganin®, Feminax®, Syndol®, Propain®, Paramol®, Migraleve®).

Tramadol (Zamadol®, Zydol®) is a new type of drug that resembles morphine, but was thought to be less addictive. It is a stronger pain medication. Small amounts of Tramadol are secreted into breastmilk. One study of 75 women (Salman et al., 2011) showed no adverse effects in breastfed infants whose mothers had taken it. As with other opiate analgesics, it is sensible to observe the baby for drowsiness, feeding difficulties, and breathing problems.

If any of these are noted, the drug should be discontinued and medical advice sought.

Antihistamines for Allergic Reactions Including Hay Fever

The Spring and Summer months can be a nightmare for people who suffer from hay fever. Breastfeeding mothers can take non-sedating antihistamines, such as Loratadine (Clarityn®), Cetirizine (Zirtek®, BecoAllergy®, Piriteze®, Benadryl®), and Fexofenadine (Telfast® Allegra®). Sedating antihistamines (those that make you drowsy) can be taken for very short courses when they may relieve the irritation of bites or an allergic rash, but long-term, they may make the mother and the baby drowsy, resulting in poor feeding and slow weight gain accompanied by a lower milk supply. These include chlorpheniramine (Piriton®, Promethazine (Phenergan®) and Trimeprazine (Vallergan®).

Steroid nasal sprays act locally, and are unlikely to pass into breastmilk in significant quantities. Corticosteroid sprays may be used to block the allergic response locally (e.g., Beclometasone (Beconase®), Fluticasone (Flixonase® Pirinase®), Budesonide (Rhinocort®), Dexa-methasone (Dexa-Rhinospray®), Mometasone (Nasonex®), and Triamcinolone (Nasocort®). Other products are designed to block the passage of pollen into the nose thus preventing the reaction (e.g., Prevalin allergy®, NasalGuard Allergic Block®), and similar own brand pharmacy products. These will not pass into breastmilk.

Eye drops also act only locally and can be used during breastfeeding (e.g., sodium cromoglycate [Opticrom®]).

Antibiotics

On a public-health level, we all try to use antibiotics only when essential. A breastfeeding mother can use antibiotics and carry on breastfeeding the baby as normal. Most antibiotics can cause the baby to have runny poo and a degree of colicky belly pains. The value of continued breastfeeding outweighs the temporary inconvenience. In theory, exposure may sensitise the baby to later doses (e.g., penicillin allergy), but this is exceedingly rare.

Large doses of antibiotics may encourage overgrowth of thrush (Candida) in the mother by killing all the natural gut bacteria. Many women find taking supplements of acidophilus or live yoghurt beneficial to redress the balance. Breastmilk contains all the factors necessary to restore the gut balance in the baby, and baby probiotics are not necessary.

The following antibiotics are all safe to take while breastfeeding.

- Amoxycillin (Amoxil®)
- Azithromycin (Zithromax®, Zmax®)
- Cefaclor (Distaclor® Ceclor®)
- Cefuroxamine (Zinnat®, Zinacef®)
- Cephalexin / Cefalexin, (Keflex®)
- Cephradine (Velosef®)
- Clarithromycin (Klaricid®, Biaxin®)
- Co-amoxiclav (Augmentin®)
- Co-fluampicil, Flucloxacillin + Ampicillin (Magnapen®)
- Erythromycin (Erymax®, Erythrope®, Erythrocin®, Eryped®)
- Flucloxacillin (Floxapen®)
- Penicillin V / Phenoxymethyl penicillin
- Trimethoprim (Monotrim®)

All are available as liquid forms to treat infant infections, and the amount getting through breastmilk is very much smaller than that which could be given to the baby directly if he was ill.

Tetracyclines were believed in the past to be contraindicated in breastfeeding because they could stain the infant's teeth (even if they had not appeared). In short courses (less than a month), this appears not to be a problem, as the drug forms a complex with the calcium in the milk, and is not absorbed by the baby. Long courses (e.g., for acne) should be avoided wherever possible. The drugs in this family are tetracycline, oxytetracycline, minocycline (Minicin®), and doxycycline (Vibramycin®).

Metronidazole (Flagyl®) has been said to impart an unpleasant taste to the milk and cause the baby to reject it. It has not been possible to trace the original research that suggested this, or who tasted the milk and made this conclusion. Babies do not appear to be concerned by the frequent variation in the taste of breastmilk that occurs naturally. Occasionally, it can alter the colour of the milk. In the U.S., single doses of 2 g are used and breastfeeding is temporarily interrupted. In the UK, doses of 200 to 400 mg three times a day are used, and breastfeeding can continue. Anecdotally, increased maternal consumption of garlic masks the taste of the metronidazole.

Ciprofloxacin (Ciproxin®) can cause problems in the joints of juvenile animals given it directly. The relevance to breastfeeding is unknown, and while short maternal courses are unlikely to pose problems, other antibiotics are preferable (e.g., trimethoprim or nitrofurantoin) as first line for simple urinary tract infections. It is not a reason to stop breastfeeding.

Nitrofurantoin (Furadantin®, Macrodantin®, Macrobid®) is excreted into breastmilk in small amounts, but may cause haemolysis in G6PD deficient infants (a comparatively rare condition involving enzyme deficiency). It may colour the mother's urine, tears, and milk yellow. This is not significant, and mothers can continue to breastfeed as normal.

Vancomycin and teicoplanin (Vancocin® and Targocid®) are used to treat multiple resistant staphylococcus aureus (MRSA). The side effects of these drugs are potentially severe, and their use requires blood counts, and kidney and liver function tests. Use to treat MRSA is generally by intravenous and intramuscular absorption. Oral absorption is poor, but there is little information on use in lactation, or studies of milk transfer. The mother may not feel well enough to breastfeed during therapy, but if she feels well enough, these drugs are not a contraindication.

Topical anti-infective creams, ointments and gels are not sufficiently absorbed to pass into breastmilk. If they are applied to the nipple, any visible product should be gently wiped off prior to breastfeeding (e.g., fusidic acid (Fucidin®) and mupirocin (Bactroban®)).

Cold Remedies

Most of us catch coughs and colds during the winter and want to feel better as soon as possible. The worst symptom is usually a runny or bunged-up nose. Breastfeeding mothers can take Paracetamol and/or ibuprofen to relieve symptoms, but should avoid decongestants, such as pseudoephedrine and phenylephrine, as a single dose of these can reduce milk supply by 24% (Aljazaf et al., 2003). Inhaling steam is a simple really usefully remedy. Products, such as menthol, or proprietary products, such as Vicks® and Olbas Oil® can be added too. However, do not apply products, such as Vick's Vap-o Rub, to the mother's chest as menthol can be toxic to babies.

Sore Throats

Sore throats can be relieved by the use of throat sprays and gargles, or by sucking lozenges, which do not get into breastmilk. Branded examples include Difflam Throat Spray or Gargle®, Chloraseptic®, Strepsils®, Dequadin®, and Tyrozets®

Cough Mixtures/Linctus

Cough linctus to soothe tickly coughs can be taken so long as they do not contain an antihistamine, which may cause drowsiness in the mum and baby. Expectorant mixtures containing guaifenesin can be taken by breastfeeding mothers to relieve a chesty cough. Avoid a multi-ingredient cough and cold mixture, as this will probably contain a decongestant.

Constipation

Constipation has been described as the fourth stage of labour. It is not uncommon after childbirth. It can be caused by pain medications. However, the sheer thought of a bowel motion after delivery and stitches can make a woman put off going until she becomes constipated. Yes, I know this isn't a topic which we discuss with our loved ones, but seriously, you have probably seen more of her personal areas in the past few days in ways than you ever dreamed. So maybe just now you could discuss it, or just leave this book open at this page in the loo?

There are medicines that can bulk and soften stools, making them easier to pass (e.g., lactulose, magnesium hydroxide, and a variety of granules added to water). It is also important that the new mum drinks plenty of fluids, and not just tea and coffee, which can be constipating in themselves.

Other things that can help are to not avoid the urge "to go"—not always easy with a new baby if you are in the middle of breast-feeding! We all know that lots of fruit and vegetables are good and help to prevent constipation. Sadly, there are a lot of old wives' tales that too much fruit will upset the baby, and that vegetables give babies wind. Not true! Different babies respond to different foods, but there is no reason to avoid the natural goodness of fruits and vegetables, and they can help you avoid constipation.

Contraception

Mothers who are exclusively breastfeeding are unlikely to ovulate, and may not have periods return for some months. Some people use this as a method of natural contraception.

The Lactational Amenorrhoea Method (LAM) is over 98% effective in preventing pregnancy if ALL of the following factors apply:

- ◉ The mother is fully breastfeeding not giving the baby any other liquid or solid food,
- ◉ The baby is less than 6 months old,
- ◉ And the mother has not resumed menstruation.

You need to be aware that if you are using this method, you should be aware that the risk of pregnancy is increased if breastfeeding decreases (particularly night feeds).

Other non-hormonal methods of contraception include use of condoms, the diaphragm, or a copper coil.

Hormonal contraceptive while breastfeeding. Choose a progesterone-only pill (mini-pill) after discussion with GP or family planning nurse. These are usually started at or after the 6-week postnatal check.

Use of progesterone-only methods while breastfeeding provides over 99% effectiveness. Irregular bleeding may be associated with this method of contraception, and it is important that you are aware of the need to take your medication regularly, and what to do if you suffer from vomiting or diarrhoea.

Hormonal implant. Anecdotally, some women note that their milk supply diminishes when they start progesterone-only products. It is worth trying one month of oral medication before starting a hormonal implant, such as depo.

Mirena® coil. This is a coil that also releases small amounts of progestogen hormone into the womb. It is 99% effective, and is claimed to be particularly useful for women having heavy periods. It is probably better to only use if there is no reduction in supply after trying the mini pill. It is left in place for 3 to 5 years.

The combined contraceptive pill. Although in theory, this is suitable after milk supply is well established, in practice, the estrogen content often reduces supply dramatically, so avoid if possible.

Barrier methods. Condoms, caps, the simple copper coil etc. are suitable during breastfeeding, but may need additional lubrication in the early postnatal period.

Stomach Bugs Including Norovirus (Winter Vomiting Bug)

The number of cases of vomiting and diarrhoea seems to increase. When a breastfeeding mother contracts a stomach bug, she may be worried about passing on the infection to her baby via the breastmilk. In fact, her milk contains antibodies to help to protect the baby. It doesn't mean the baby won't get the bug, but if he does, he will probably have it less severely. Exclusively breastfed babies are less likely to catch any gastrointestinal bugs than those fed with formula milk.

You may purchase, or the mum may be prescribed drugs to help relieve the vomiting (e.g., prochloperazine (Stemetil®, Buccastem®) or promethazine (Phenergan®)). She may need loperamide (Imodium®, Imodium plus®, Imodium instant®) to stop the diarrhoea. If she can manage, it is better to let the body expel the bug via the diarrhoea, but this may not always be possible. In order to avoid dehydration, keep on sipping water or rehydration solution (Dioralyte®). If possible, the mum should keep on breastfeeding as normal, but have the baby cared for by another adult. That's you, Dad and Grandma, as you keep providing her with drinks and simple foods as she recovers. Keep washing your hands in hot, soapy water, and disinfect the loo so that, hopefully, you don't catch it.

Vitamin D Deficiency

UK Guidelines are that mothers should continue to take vitamin D during breastfeeding, and to give supplementary drops to babies after they reach the age of 6 months. The American Academy of Pediatrics (Wagner & Greer, 2008 http://pediatrics.aappublications.org/content/122/5/1142.short) recommend a daily intake of vitamin D of 10 mg (400 IU/day) for all infants and children beginning in the first few days of life.

Hollis and colleagues (2015) showed that supplementation with 6400 IU is necessary to significantly increased maternal vitamin D and 25(OH)D from baseline, and reduce the need for direct supplementation for the infant.

Why is it Necessary to Take Vitamin D Supplements?

The incidence of rickets in children is increasing again after becoming very rare following supplementation of most children with cod liver oil after the Second World War. One reason is the concerns about sunburn and the risk of skin cancer. Most children (and adults) wear a high-factor sunscreen whenever they are in the sun (and rightly so. There is no excuse for allowing a child to be sunburned), but it limits the vitamin D produced naturally by the body. Vitamin D is also contained in foods, such as oily fish. Oily fish include trout, salmon, mackerel, herring, sardines, anchovies, pilchards, and fresh tuna. Other sources of vitamin D are egg yolk, some cereals, dairy spreads, and mushrooms. These are not everyone's favourites.

Many adults are now vitamin D deficient between October and April, and many will have low levels throughout the year. Anybody living north of the latitude of Birmingham (UK) is also unlikely to be exposed to sufficient ultraviolet radiation to produce vitamin D in the summer, let alone the winter. A map of the equivalent U.S. map is shown here. Mothers should all take vitamin D throughout pregnancy to ensure that the baby has adequate levels at birth. Babies born to mothers with low vitamin D status are at risk of developing rickets. If she has not taken vitamin D prior to pregnancy, even if she begins to take a supplement herself after delivery, she cannot redress the baby's deficiency by breastfeeding alone. So the recommendation in this case is that the baby should receive its own oral vitamin D drops containing 7.5 microgrammes (300 IU) per day from 4 weeks after birth until the age of 5 years. This doesn't mean that breastmilk isn't perfect, just that our modern life has altered our body's ability to do what it can do naturally. If the mum has taken supplements in pregnancy, the baby doesn't need to begin drops until 6 months.

People who are not exposed to much sun, such as those who cover up for cultural reasons or who have darker skin, such as those of African, African-Caribbean, and South Asian origin are more prone to vitamin D deficiency.

Medical Procedures

Operations

If your partner needs to have an operation while she is breast-feeding, there is no reason to interrupt breastfeeding. The drugs used in anaesthetics stay in the body a very short length of time, which is why you are awake so quickly. Some drug gets stored in the fat cells of her body (and even the slimmest of us have fat cells). This is slowly released over the following 24 hours, and at worst, she and your baby may feel a bit drowsy. If she is staying in hospital, you may need to negotiate how to keep the baby with her, perhaps in a single room, or if this is not possible, access to a breast pump and somewhere to store the milk. It may be that you or Grandma can look after your baby nearby, and bring him in to be breastfed, or you can sleep in a chair beside her bed.

Dental Treatment

Breastfeeding mothers can have fillings, local anaesthetics, teeth out, use mouth washes, have tooth whitening, and have treatment under sedation without changing breastfeeding at all. Sedation usually involves the drug midazolam (Hypnovel®, Versed®), which stays in the body for a short space of time and shouldn't affect the baby at all, even if it is breastfed straight after the procedure.

MRI Scans

It seems increasingly common for MRI and CT scans to be used as diagnostic tools. These may or may not involve the use of contrast media. Radiographers may well suggest that a mother cannot breastfeed for 24 hours after use of such products. It is not radioactive, and is given by intravenous injection into the arm. The gadolinium will be excreted (removed) from the body through the kidneys within 24 hours. For this reason, it is often suggested that mothers should pump and dump their breastmilk during this time.

There is no need to discontinue breastfeeding after the contrast medium has been given, or to pump to clear milk of the contrast medium (Goergen & Molan, 2009). The amount that will pass to the baby is very small and does not represent a risk. Oral absorption is minimal, with only 0.8% of gadopentetate being absorbed (American College of Radiology Committee on Drugs and Contrast Media, 2010; Chen et al., 2008; Hale & Rowe, 2014; Lactmed, 2016; Webb et al., 2015).

The concerns of radiologists to avoid exposing any baby to any product is understandable, but dismisses the needs of the mother and baby to continue breastfeeding. Expressing for 24 hours after the procedure is not without difficulty. The use of artificial formula milk is not without risks, and some babies refuse to feed from a bottle, whether given expressed breastmilk or formula milk.

Colonoscopy

I frequently get asked about the safety of colonoscopies and endoscopies for breastfeeding mothers. These may be for mothers with the chronic conditions Crohn's Disease and Colitis, with symptoms of gastric pain suggesting ulcers, or to rule out any serious condition.

The procedures usually involve cleansing of the gut using strong laxatives and a low residue diet over the 24 hours before the procedure. The products normally used contain laxatives that pull water into the gut, and are not absorbed into breastmilk. During this period, the mother may only be allowed to drink clear fluids and not eat. It is important that she drinks freely during this period if she is breastfeeding in order to prevent diarrhoea. She will have frequent bowel motions, which will become increasingly liquid as the gut is washed out. She won't be moving far from the toilet, so you may need to stay close to take over the baby while she attends to her own needs. Trust me, this is not the time to try breastfeeding on the toilet!

Before the procedure, the mother will be given sedatives to relax her and induce a light sleep. These normally include pethidine, midazolam, and fentanyl. These drugs all have very short half-lives (the periods they stay in the body). The mum will be wide awake and able to leave hospital very shortly after the procedure, and can feed as soon as she gets home.

Resuming Sex

Grandma, please feel free to miss out on reading this section!

When you decide to resume sex is a decision for the two of you. Some couples don't wait very long, while others find themselves months after the birth still not having an intimate relationship, as they are too tired by the demands of a new baby, or have found it too painful.

For some women, the pain of stitches does not go as soon as they expect. It can be painful to sit down, let alone consider intercourse. For others, there is no issue. Most health care professionals suggest that penetrative sex is not resumed until after the 6-week postnatal check to prevent infection. The cervix does not close immediately and uterine infections can occur.

When you decide the time is right for you, take your time and be aware that your little bundle may choose that moment to wake up, so you need to keep a sense of humour. You may need additional lubrication creams and remember, even if your partner hasn't had a return of periods, you need to use contraception if the baby is more than 6 months old. If the baby is less than 6 months, is being exclusively breastfed with no long periods between feeds (day and night), and your partner has not had a period, there is a 98% effectiveness that lactational amenorrhoea will prevent pregnancy without the need for contraception (The Family Planning Association www.fpa.org.uk/home).

Contraceptive choices during breastfeeding are the progester-one-only (mini pill) contraceptive: tablet, depo injection, implant or coil, simple IUD, barrier methods, but not the combined oral contraceptive. See earlier section on contraceptives.

If your partner is still finding that her scar from her perineal stitches is still sore after 3 months, she should discuss this with her GP. In some cases, oestrogen cream is advised to help healing. In theory, absorption of these should not be sufficient to affect breastmilk supply. However, anecdotally, some mothers do notice a drop in milk production. This is a time when, as a loving partner, you may need to consider how to satisfy everyone's needs and use your imagination!

What Happens if the Mum Gets Pregnant While Still Breastfeeding?

Sometimes parents rely on natural contraception when the baby is over 6 months of age, or just forget to use contraception, and a pregnancy results. You might also not be actively using contraception, and not be worried about another pregnancy. If you are happy for the pregnancy to continue, that is brilliant. You do not need to stop breastfeeding the nursling. Many mothers go on to tandem breastfeed, while others give up because they find that their nipples are painful in early pregnancy, or when their milk supply dwindles in pregnancy. There is no need to stop to prevent a risk of miscarriage. When milk is released, oxytocin is produced, as we have already discussed. This hormone makes the womb contract, but does not put the new baby at risk unless the pregnancy is already very unstable and likely to miscarry anyway. How and when you decide to wean is your choice, but you may encounter surprise from people who have never considered breastfeeding while pregnant.

If, however, you decide that you need to terminate the pregnancy, or your partner miscarries, she can continue to breastfeed your other child. There are surgical and medical options that can be discussed with your health care professionals.

Breastfeeding When the Mother has a Chronic Medical Condition

Many people assume that if they have a chronic medical condition necessitating the use of ongoing medication that they will not be able to breastfeed. This is rarely true. There are usually options. However, again I need to stress that if you decide, as a family, that breastfeeding is no longer the best for you, then it is fine to stop. I am hoping to present options, not pressure.

I am going to discuss some of the conditions I get asked about most frequently. This isn't a definitive list, but again, this isn't a book about breastfeeding and illness.

Asthma

We have already discussed that breastfeeding protects against asthma to a degree. That isn't to say that everyone with asthma was fed exclusively with formula milk, or that exclusive breastfeeding will prevent your child from getting any symptoms. These data are based on population studies that show a benefit of breastfeeding for a minimum of 4 months. If you are interested in looking at the studies, you will find them here: www.unicef.org.uk/BabyFriendly/News-and-Research/Research/Asthma/.

Inhalers form the mainstay of asthma prevention and treatment. These act locally in the lungs, and do not reach significant levels in breastmilk. Reliever inhaler (blue inhalers), such as salbutamol/albuterol (Ventolin®), and preventer inhalers (brown), such as beclometasone (Becotide®), or the dual action ones, such as Seretide®, do not require any change in breastfeeding.

Steroids may be required during a flare of symptoms, or along-side antibiotics. Doses of up to 40 mg prednisolone can be taken during breastfeeding without negatively affecting the baby.

Monteleukast (Singulair®) does not have any research on how much gets into breastmilk, but we give it directly to babies with asthma from 6 months of age. It is often given to people with severe season allergies, as well as asthma.

Crohn's and Ulcerative Colitis

I will share with you that I personally have Crohn's disease, and have had to have 3 bowel resections since my diagnosis at the age of 22 years. My symptoms are managed with medication. I was lucky in that my children were all born at times when I was symptom free, so I did not have to breastfeed on medication. However, I would never say anything is "safe" if I would not have taken it myself. Those of us with inflammatory bowel disease pass on a genetic predisposition to our children to develop the condition. It is also to some degree linked with being formula-fed as a child. So we have every reason to breastfeed, and continue with our medication. Some mothers apparently stop their drugs in order to breastfeed, and then experience a flare of symptoms. I was never fitter than when I was pregnant and breastfeeding, which led me to my passion for breastfeeding, and ultimately, this book.

Azathioprine (Imuran®) is an immuno-suppressant often used particularly to maintain remission after steroids have got symptoms under control. Taking it means regular blood tests to monitor cell counts. This means that it is often regarded with some caution in the breastfeeding mother. In fact, the amount getting through breastmilk is small, so babies do not need monitoring, and breastfeeding can continue as normal.

Steroids can be necessary to reduce symptoms of a flare-up. Doses of 40 mg a day of prednisolone can safely be taken during breastfeeding, slightly higher doses short-term.

Cytokine modulators. There are lots of drugs given when tablets don't work to dampen down the inflammation. These include infliximab (Remicade®), adalimumab (Humira®), and golimumab (Simponi®). The research on these varies, but in general, they are high molecular weight, poorly bio-available drugs (don't get absorbed from the gut so have to be given by injection/infusion), so in theory the baby will not absorb the drug.

Sulphasalazine (Salazopyrin®) **and mesalazine** (Asacol®, Pentasa®) are also used in breastfeeding with rare reports of diarrhoea (not breastfed bowel motions).

Rheumatoid Arthritis

This is a chronic inflammation causing pain and stiffness in joints. In some people, it can be managed by anti-inflammatory drugs, such as ibuprofen, diclofenac, and naproxen (possibly with omeprazole to protect the stomach). These can be taken long-term by breast-feeding mothers. Other drugs prescribed include sulphasalazine and hydroxychloroquine (Plaquenil®), which can be taken during breastfeeding. The use of the stronger disease modifying agent methotrexate is more problematic. Research in 2014 suggests that it may, however, be possible to breastfeed, although this is based on just one case report (Thorne et al., 2014). Hale and Rowe recommend pumping and dumping for 24 hours after once-weekly therapy (Hale & Rowe, 2014). Biological treatments are a newer form of treatment for rheumatoid arthritis. They include etanercept, infliximab, adalimumab, golimumab, and rituximab. As in IBD, the safety is based largely on theoretical data. For more information, have a look at the research that breastfeeding helps protect the mother from developing rheumatoid arthritis: www.unicef.org.uk/BabyFriendly/News-and-Research/Research/Rheumatoid-arthritis/.

Diabetes

Mothers who are type 1, insulin-dependent diabetics can breast-feed. Insulin is not absorbed orally by the baby via breastmilk. Usually breastfeeding mothers can eat more carbohydrate for the same dose of insulin, or decrease insulin requirements. It is essential to keep healthy snacks available, particularly overnight. As we know, breastfeeding is protective against insulin-dependent diabetes, it is another reason to avoid formula milk. For more information, have a look at the research: www.unicef.org.uk/BabyFriendly/News-and-Research/Research/Diabetes/.

CONCLUSION

Dad and Grandma, your role in supporting the new mother in your family is indescribably important. She and her new baby rely on you to be there for them during the long nights and early mornings, to be a source of comfort during the confusing maybe painful times, to help her make decisions (based on evidence, not on the advice of others, however well-meaning, or the results of random Google searches), and maybe to assist in solving problems.

The breastfeeding journey for your new family may be straight-forward, or it may not be. Take each day at a time. Every day of breastfeeding is important. Tell your partner or daughter what a great job she is doing, and treasure her.

I hope that this book provides you with information on which to make the choices you need, whether it is that you need to phone a friend, call the doctor, or buy a take out because you are all tired. Breastfeeding is the best way to feed your baby, and that is why you have bought this book. But it is something that may take time and effort to achieve.

Enjoy being a family. The days pass all too quickly, and soon, your little one will be grown up, and sleeping all day and up all night. It never changes!

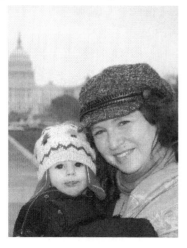
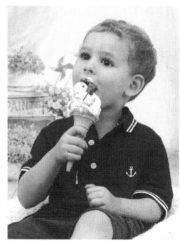

THE STORY OF CHRISTIAN, KERENSA, AND STIRLING

For me, to be part of my daughter's labour was a moving experience. I expected to be uncomfortable watching her in pain, but in fact, it felt like watching her blossom gradually over that day into motherhood. We spent a momentous hour walking together in the early morning. We met a woman out walking her dogs. She recognised 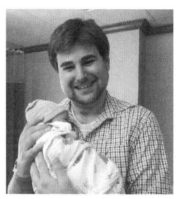 what was going on and empathised with us: the joining of women to embrace labour. Did you know that the term "midwife" means "with woman," and they weren't always highly trained professionals, but maybe just the village elders?

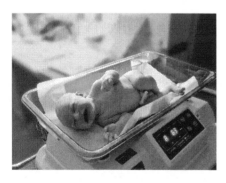 I was also so privileged to be present throughout the second stage of labour, and watched my precious grandson emerge into the world, delivered onto his mother's chest by his adoring father. This was a moment that will be etched into my mind for the rest of my life. I watched the transformation of my daughter's face from the pain of birth to ecstasy as she took in the first sight, touch, and smell of her son.

As my daughter found out, the priority after her baby was born seemed to be to weigh the baby, suck out any mucus remaining, administer a hepatitis B injection, and then for a professional to attach the baby to the breast. I have a photograph in which you can clearly see the distress on his face as he startles under the lights of the cot in which he is placed. Sadly, I was busy taking pictures.

The picture of the first feed my daughter and grandson shared clearly showed the gloved hand of a health care professional who arrived to facilitate. The baby was already dressed in a nappy and hat. He was also lightly swaddled. You can also see the hand behind the baby's head and the pressure on the breast. Both would be unnecessary if they had been left in skin to skin.

Baby Stirling attached for his very first breastfeed with gusto and enthusiasm. It was as if he had read all the books and articles that have been part of my breastfeeding world over the past 26 years.

The hospital not only permitted, but expected the dad to stay with his new family. A bed was available in the room, so my daughter had help with changing nappies, getting iced drinks, and being supported through the night. I clearly remember feeling very lonely when I was left by myself on the ward after the delivery of my babies. The responsibility was huge, especially when coupled with the discomfort of stitches. Grandad and I left the new family for the night, after taking lots of photographs!

Our First Day After Birth

We returned the following morning in time to attend the breastfeeding class held daily on the ward by one of the lactation consultants. We listened to an excellent discussion on how breastfeeding works, what to look for, and when to call for help. We were also given a simple, but excellent booklet called *Better Breastfeeding*. It contained lots of photographs, simple texts, and links to further information. My daughter had no particular concerns, but listened closely – I'm sure just checking that I was saying the right things. The lactation consultant also provided individual support during the inpatient stay, and was available after, but with a charge. This is different from the UK, where mothers continue to see health care professionals, such as midwives, free of charge, although they can choose to see an IBCLC.

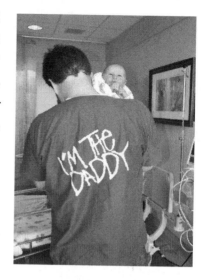

In his first full day of life, my grandson was a very drowsy baby, unwilling to attach with an open mouth, and with a definite preference for one side. It was all totally normal and not unexpected. Sleep is nature's way of allowing everyone a breather after the hectic labour-day.

His initial latch was often painful for my daughter. We could improve it, but certainly not make it totally comfortable at every feed. I wanted my "magic wand." Having not helped many mothers face-to-face for many years, although I knew most theories, this was very hard for me and confusing for everyone else. On one breast, it seemed easier to use a rugby hold with the baby's legs under Mum's arm. It was easier to move his hands from his face, although the right hand was still close, but not impeding attachment!

163

Our Second Night in Hospital

In her large single room, my daughter could call a member of staff to support her with breastfeeding at any time. They checked on her feeding and said that everything looked fine, despite the fact that she was experiencing pain.

I spent the second night in hospital with my daughter, leaving Christian to get a good night's sleep. My husband had left for the airport, as he had to fly back to the UK. Luckily, he had been able to spend 24 hours with our new grandson.

The baby woke to feed every couple of hours, and seemed to settle reasonably well after feeding. Upon changing his nappy, I noticed that his urine was a salmon pink colour, which the nurse confirmed was due to the passage of uric acid. This suggests that his fluid intake was not as good as it should be. However, we were reassured that all looked well, and we should keep making sure that he breastfed every 2 hours, and not to allow him to sleep for more than 4 hours.

I remained concerned, as I felt that his attachment wasn't perfect as my daughter continued to experience pain. Although it eased during the feed, it didn't go completely. It was a continual struggle to convince him to keep his hands away from his face—a position that we had seen him adopt in scans.

The following morning, the new baby was examined again by the hospital paediatrician, pronounced fit and well, and ready for discharge. He was, however, slightly jaundiced, and they requested that he see his own paediatrician the following day. The salmon-pink uric acid crystal-stained nappies were dismissed, and my daughter was told she did not need to wake him to feed. That was something I was not sure was good information, but thought it was unlikely that he would sleep that long anyway. I wanted to see him feed frequently and effectively until I saw plenty of wet nappies (without colour), and nice yellow poo, rather than the dark green meconium we were still seeing. I wasn't going to relax.

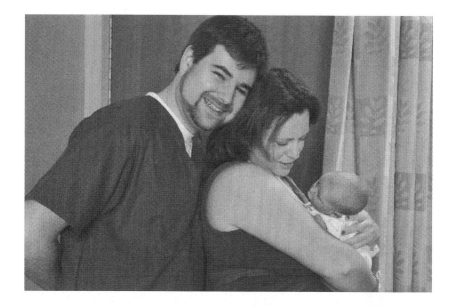

Home!

When my grandson first came home after birth, his father was keen to settle him between feeds. Somehow, the baby would not stop crying, but would calm instantly in my arms.

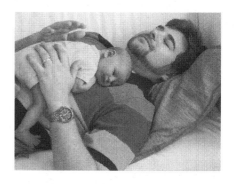

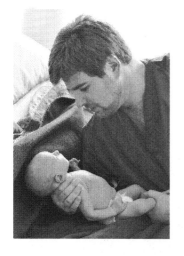

This was a source of great frustration to my son-in-law (and me, as I didn't want to interfere in the bonding process). Was it because he sensed that I was an old hand with babies? Was I trying less hard? When I watched it, became apparent that Christian would hold the baby with his own arms outstretched (partly because he was farsighted, but also to look at the baby), so Stirling felt vulnerable and continued cry.

When cuddled in close, he settled and went to sleep on Christian's chest, giving Mum some much needed time to sleep, and his dad a wonderful time to gaze at his son, enjoying skin to skin.

At home, we found a position that felt comfortable and facilitated a good breastfeed; the mum's arm straight down her side, the baby's head resting along arm, and breast supported, but not shaped. The mum supported on pillows, with encouragement from a very proud dad.

In view of the jaundice, we were advised to see the baby's own paediatrician at the offices 24 hours after discharge to monitor his weight. This showed that at day 3, his weight was still dropping, but on day 4, had stabilised despite the ongoing uric acid crystals, and infrequent green poo. No one seemed concerned except me. As a family, we decided to visit the lactation consultant associated with the hospital. We saw her on day 5, and saw a small, but significant weight increase with improved output, as depicted by the wee and poo chart. On day 6, at the paediatrician's office, we saw the first significant increase in weight. Throughout, no one suggested topping up with formula milk, and encouraged exclusive breastfeeding.

At the visit to the lactation consultant, my daughter achieved a pain-free latch at last, and the baby fed contentedly for some 40 minutes. He wasn't interested in feeding from the second side. He was full and contented. So all was well, wasn't it?

The lactation consultant had suggested the cross-cradle rather than cradle hold, and had given my daughter a much flatter breast-feeding pillow that could be attached around her waist, keeping it in place. She had also noticed, as I had done on the second day of his life, that he didn't bring his tongue forward to cover his lips. He was willing to suck your finger only if it was far back in his mouth. I had spent some time getting him to accept just the fingertip into his mouth to elicit a suck, and assumed the problem was resolved.

The lactation consultant termed it "snap back." I had visions of tongue-tie snipping (frenulotomy). The very first thing I checked when holding him was that he didn't have a tongue-tie; he could move his tongue upwards and sideways. So I was concerned. I had recently heard a paediatrician say that a ridge at the back of the tongue is palpable in many new babies. I tensed, but no mention was made of snipping. He fed well without causing pain, after some attention to positioning and attachment, so I relaxed.

I was interested that the baby was also test-weighed; weighed in just a nappy before and after a breastfeed. My daughter found this reassuring because there was good milk transfer, but it could have been devastating if this had not been the case. However, it would also have been indicative that whatever we were seeing, the baby might not be actively breastfeeding, or the mother's milk supply might be compromised. As a single measurement, I would not recommend it, but as part of a full assessment, it was useful with emphasis on the frequency of wet and dirty nappies being emphasised.

At home, we could not replicate the totally pain-free feeding. We looked at the close up photographs we had taken to check where hands and arms were placed, and where the baby was positioned with respect to the nipple. The pain wasn't awful, and there was no major nipple trauma; just a slight grazing. I remained worried as the poo in the nappies was still greener than I wanted to see, and not frequent enough to reassure me.

My daughter decided to order the different breastfeeding pillow; her current one was thick and placed the baby too high. It also tended to spring out however we placed it. My son-in-law commented on the chair in which she generally sat to feed. It didn't allow her to sit upright with her back supported. We settled on using a computer chair with her feet supported on, at first, a pile of books, then a wooden stool to enable her to have a flat lap.

Success! With the new pillow, and a rolled-up blanket popped behind the shoulders of the baby, we got pain-free breastfeeding, and the nappies turned bright yellow, and became very frequent. Better still, on day 10, the weight was going back up. Hallelujah!

We often expect that babies alert us to their needs by crying. In fact, as far as feeding cues go, crying comes in very late. If you watch your baby, you will notice a lot of body language much earlier. Feeding at this point ensures frequent effective feeding. What is not helpful is for Dad or Grandma to try to keep the baby away from Mum, delaying breastfeeds. Babies need feeding at least 12 times a day, and sometimes even more often. Following the baby's lead is important in establishing and maintaining a good milk supply. Letting the baby cry will actually make breast-feeding harder, as the baby will be more difficult to attach. It is usually upsetting for everyone as well. Hearing a baby in distress is uncomfortable.

First Trip Out and Feeding in Public

After 3 weeks, with everything looking good, my daughter and I went along to the local La Leche League group meeting. Peer-sup-port organisations are less common in the U.S. than in the UK, where you may be able to access others mothers trained by the Breastfeeding Network, The National Childbirth Trust, The Associ-ation of Breastfeeding Mothers, and La Leche League. The group we attended is held in the cafe of a wholefood supermarket. I did not really know what to expect. Would it be like our local drop in groups? Would it be one-to-one support or a social group? It was to be held at 10 a.m., and involved a half-hour drive, so we were up early and organised; no mean feat at that time, still.

We found the group quite easily, mainly due to the obvious copy of the *Womanly Art of Breastfeeding* on the table – good hint! There were 4 other people around a table, and they moved out to give us space to join. I left my daughter to introduce herself, and went to buy drinks for us.

I sat back, watched, and listened. There was a La Leche leader there, who I later discovered worked in a local hospital too, another mother with her 4-week-old baby, and two mums due shortly, and on the same day. The pregnant mums raised many of the questions we hear in peer-support groups everywhere, generally needing reassurance as they started to think beyond the birth. The mother with the 4-week-old was feeding confidently, using a fine silk scarf to lightly cover her breasts.

My grandson soon woke up and started to exhibit feeding cues. I wondered what was in my daughter's mind. This was the first breastfeed outside of the home. I helped her drape her sling across her shoulder to cover her breast discreetly, but rapidly, it became apparent that she wasn't that worried. By the time we got to the second side and back again, it was barely in use as she chatted happily to the others. Brilliant – the most useful outcome of a peer-support group was confidence to breastfeed outside the home. Other people walked through the coffee area, but none paid any attention to the feeding group; just a few smiles at the tiny babies.

The second good outcome of the group was that the mother of the 4-week-old talked about the problems that she had had: she had needed nipple creams for soreness, but that around 3 weeks, it had suddenly all resolved. Lots of realism, but also positivity for the others.

After the others left, we loitered for my daughter to discuss a few points where she needed encouragement and affirmation from someone other than me. We talked about breastfeeding support in the UK and U.S. We also discussed a drug that my daughter had received during her postnatal haemorrhage. It appeared that in some local hospitals, mothers are not allowed to breastfeed for 12 hours after receiving it. I promised to undertake some research to support mothers to be able to continue breastfeeding, as my daughter had done. I wondered what I would have done if she had been told not to breastfeed after its use, with me being an "expert" on the passage of drugs in breastmilk. I couldn't bear thinking about it.

The Following Weeks

I had to return to the UK shortly after the LLL meeting, and left the new family unit happily settled into their new life. Grandma and Grandpa Klottrup were going out to spend a month with the family, so there would be lots of support.

The weather in the U.S. was hot, so my daughter spent lots of time in the air-conditioned basement rooms. I had reassured her that despite the heat, the baby would need no extra fluids because breastmilk provides everything.

The Sad Times

The new little family spent just 3 weeks by themselves before Christian became suddenly ill with stomach pains and vomiting.

He had been very tired over the previous 6 weeks, but this could have been explained by the inevitable lack of sleep with a new baby. He had a pain in his right side, but nothing specific. Just before Stirling was born, he had run two half-marathons, but now struggled to run for half an hour.

After a night of intense pain and severe vomiting, they decided to go to the emergency room of their local hospital. In typical Christian fashion, he insisted that they keep an appointment to get Stirling's first passport ready for the booked trip back to the UK for my second daughter's wedding.

I was kept informed during the day of the tests and results with increasing incredulity. At 7 a.m., I heard the terrible news that he had been diagnosed with metastatic colon cancer. He was due to have surgery the following day to resolve the blockage that had resulted from one rapidly growing tumour. He had a colostomy 2 days before his 35th birthday. I flew back out to Washington DC 3 days later to help with looking after them all. Kerensa and Stirling were spending all of their time at hospital.

Christian was on a drip and an epidural, as well as injected medication, to deal with breakthrough pain. He looked remarkably well, taking the diagnosis into consideration. However, each day brought more bad news. His liver was infiltrated by several tumours, and there was further spread to the lungs. The medical team wanted to scan his bones, but needed to get him comfortable enough to undertake the tests. He struggled to get up and walk as much as he could, but was very weak.

At that time, we were sleeping at home for a few hours each night, but that was soon to end. Six days after his operation, he developed pneumonia and thrombosis in his lungs. He was desperately ill. For a while, we thought he also had *C. difficile,* and he was barrier nursed. I spent my days in the family room with Stirling, popping out to the nearby supermarket to shop for food for Kerensa and me. I bought plates, cups, and cutlery in a strange attempt to keep life "normal," when it was anything but. Kerensa came out to breastfeed Stirling at regular intervals, and I can honestly say that he never cried, unlike me.

Christian's mum flew out to be with us, to be followed 2 days later by his father and brother. It was the darkest time. Each day, the tests fluctuated. One moment our hearts were up, only to plummet again. We took Christian out into the garden in a wheelchair sometimes. The ward had a beautiful healing garden with benches, water features, and a wonderful sense of peace. Stirling and I sat out there often.

Christian's mum took it in turns with us to sleep in his room which, just like the maternity unit, had a pull out bed. We went home to shower and change, eating most meals together in the family room.

After 3 weeks, I had to return to the UK to speak at a long-arranged conference, and to prepare for my daughter, Beth's, wedding. I had arranged to return within 4 weeks, after the celebrations were over. Little did I know that when I left, I would not see Christian again.

Christian was given a course of chemotherapy in a last-ditch attempt to prolong his life. All pretence of "cure" had gone, but we all prayed that it would relieve some very distressing symptoms, and enable him to enjoy some more precious time with his family. Sadly, it wasn't to be. The chemotherapy weakened his body further, and it became apparent that his situation was rapidly becoming terminal.

The family decided to arrange for Stirling to be Christened in the family room by the minister of the Church Kerensa and I had attended whenever we could. The staff transformed the room, spending their free time cleaning and rearranging it. Every attempt was made to have Christian pain-free, but conscious for the ceremony. Food and drink were purchased, and wonderful family friends, Godparents, and all of Christian's four siblings came. We had a Skype link set up from the UK, but at the last moment, it failed, and we were unable to see the Christening. Christian's bed was wheeled in, and he was fully involved in this special moment.

Tragically, just 36 hours later, he lost his battle for life, dying peacefully, surrounded by his wife, his parents, and his brothers and sisters. Stirling was nearby with a family friend. During his last days, he commented that he had no regrets, as he had packed so

171

much into his 35 years of life. It is tragic that he had just 3 and a half months with his son.

Throughout all of these distressing times, Kerensa continued to breastfeed. She had an abundant supply of breastmilk. The only way that we could explain this was that the love which she and Christian shared was so strong that oxytocin was flowing between them in the room. It was, in many ways, a peaceful room, full of people sharing a love for one person, and willing him to get better. We have kept in contact with many of the people from the ward, particularly Christian's palliative care nurse, Mimi, who has become a much loved friend to all of us. We are still in contact almost 2 years later. Exclusive breastfeeding continued to the gold standard for 6 months, and then alongside a baby-led weaning diet. Despite all that she had to deal with, the nursing, distress, and grief, my daughter breastfed without hesitation.

I have presented the picture below in every talk that I have given since, as an example of the power of oxytocin and love, that the female body can continue to provide milk in the most extreme situations, that milk does not easily dry up suddenly, and that the oxytocin is very powerful. We hope this precious image will inspire others, as I hope this book does, to remember a very precious family and a wonderful young man who would have been an awesome dad.

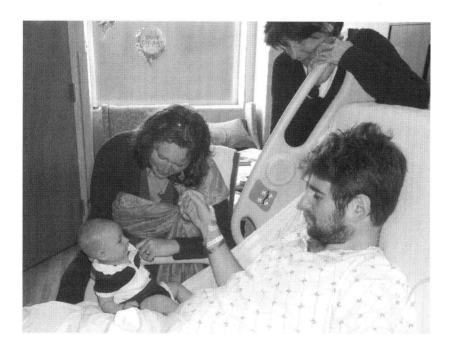

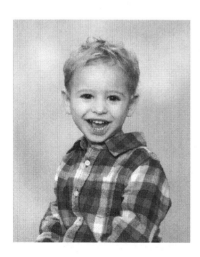

Stirling continues to grow and flourish, now back in the UK, and is currently an adorable 2-and-a-half-year-old, full of life and energy. He is still being breastfed at night, enjoying his favourite "milshies." He points to photographs of his father with delight, pronouncing "Daddy" with pride. Christian will always be his Daddy, and never be forgotten. I hope he is looking down from the stars, proud of his very special son.

A New Life

This year, another grandson came into my life. Isaac, born to my daughter Beth, whose wedding was 4 days after Christian's death. Isaac has taught me even more lessons as a grandma.

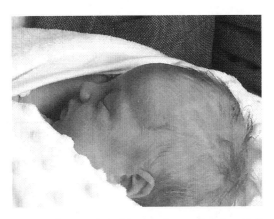

He was born 3 weeks and 1 day early, weighing 5 lbs, 10 oz. He was treated as premature for the first 24 hours in hospital. He was also born after a natural birth, at which I was again privileged to be present. He spent his first 3 hours in uninterrupted skin-to-skin contact, feeding enthusiastically in the delivery suite. On the postnatal ward, they wanted to monitor his blood sugar and temperature every 4 hours, and insisted he needed 25 ml of formula milk every 4 hours. No attempt was made to help with breastfeeding, and only after a struggle was hand expressing demonstrated by anyone other than me. We were told that if we did not agree to the formula milk, he would be admitted to SCBU and put on a drip.

I knew his stomach capacity was way below 25 ml, but felt powerless to protest at this force-feeding. We managed to negotiate that after the first volume by bottle, we could syringe and finger feed him the colostrum Beth expressed, and smaller volumes of formula milk. When she has another baby, I will make sure we have donor breastmilk available to avoid this situation. We all felt disempowered by one midwife who gave every impression of trying to undermine breastfeeding.

Within 18 hours of his birth, Isaac was breastfeeding regularly and well. By day 3, he had yellow poo, and had barely lost any weight. Apart from being dressed to drive home, he did not move from being in skin to skin with either his mum or dad for 5 days. He never did go into a hospital bassinette. He co-sleeps at home, although he has a co-sleeper available, which I am sure will one day be used other than to store clothes and nappies.

At 11 months, he weighs around 22 lb, and is chunky, relaxed, and still breastfed alongside baby-led weaning foods. So this time, we achieved skin to skin and pain-free breastfeeding from the beginning. However, we were not able to fight the top-ups in the first few hours, but accepted that this was necessary due to his prematurity. Breastfeeding has been straightforward for Beth, although the 6-week growth spurt knocked her confidence for a few days.

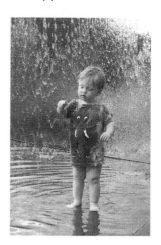

What Have I Learned This Time?

As a grandma to another precious bundle, I learned that I did have enough love for two, that no two births are the same, that no two breastfeeding experiences are the same, and that my job is to listen, support, and add knowledge when it is asked for. I also rediscovered the joy of knitting! Every moment of being a grandma is a joy to me.

As I finish this book, we are now eagerly awaiting the birth of Kerensa's new baby. She has found love again, and a partner who has been happy to share her life and Stirling's. He would be the first to admit that he will never replace Christian, but will help to raise his son with love.

Breastfeeding and the Important Others

I am lucky that my two daughters have embraced breastfeeding wholeheartedly, as have their husbands. I would support them in their choices as I support many mothers every week who ask me about the safety of drugs in breastmilk. My life is to provide evidence-based information to enable them to make choices that are right for them. I hope this book does that for every one of you who reads it, whether you are a dad, grandma, grandpa, sister, brother, best friend, or breastfeeding support worker. You are all special to a breastfeeding mother. Thank you for being there, and I hope you all enjoy your journey as the baby in your life grows.

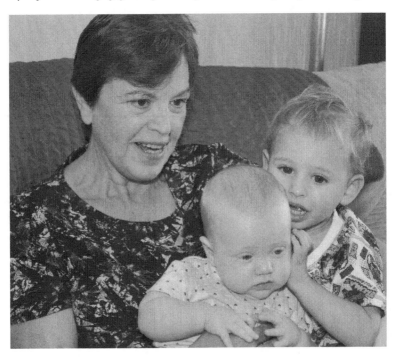

Postscript: Beatrix Mary was born at the end of June 2016, weighing 8 lb 15 oz after an emergency caesarean section for a footling breech delivery. She took to breastfeeding as a total natural, and is gaining weight beautifully. Mother and baby (as well as Dad plus Grandma and big brother Stirling) are doing well!

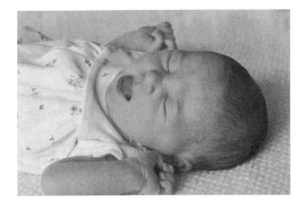

WEBSITES

- Association of Breastfeeding Mothers www.abm.me.uk
- Baby Milk Action www.babymilkaction.org
- Best Beginnings www.bestbeginnings.org.uk
- Bliss www.bliss.org.uk
- Breastfeeding and Medication www.breastfeeding-and-medication.co.uk
- The Family Planning Association www.fpa.org.uk/home
- First Steps Nutrition Trust www.firststepsnutrition.org
- Healthy Start www.healthystart.nhs.uk
- Kathy Dettwyler http://kathydettwyler.weebly.com/
- Kathleen Kendall-Tackett uppitysciencechick.com, breastfeedingmadesimple.com
- La Leche League www.laleche.org.uk
- Maternity Action www.maternityaction.org.uk
- Milk Banking Association www.ukamb.org
- Multiple Births Foundation www.multiplebirths.org.uk
- National Breastfeeding Helpline www.nationalbreastfeedinghelpline.org.uk
- National Childbirth Trust www.nct.org.uk
- NHS and breastfeeding www.nhs.uk/Conditions/pregnancy-and-baby
- NHS Start for life www.nhs.uk/start4life
- TAMBA www.tamba.org.uk
- The Breastfeeding Network www.breastfeedingnetwork.org.uk
- Tongue-Tie Practitioners www.tongue-tie.org.uk
- UNICEF Baby-Friendly Initiative www.babyfriendly.org.uk

Sources of Support

Breastfeeding helplines

- National Breastfeeding Helpline 0300-100- 0212
- Association of Breastfeeding Mothers 0300-330-5453
- The Breastfeeding Network (in English or Welsh) 0300-100-0210
    - Bengali and Sylheti: 0300-456-2421
    - Tamil, Telegu, and Hindi: 0300-330-5469
    - Drugs in Breastmilk Helpline: 0844-412-4665
- La Leche League GB 0845-120-2918
- National Childbirth Trust 0300-330-0770

REFERENCES

American College of Radiology Committee on Drugs and Contrast Media. (2010). *ACR manual on contrast media, Version 7*, 61-62.

Amitay, E.L. & Keinan-Boker, L. (2015). Breastfeeding and Childhood Leukemia Incidence: A Meta-analysis and Systematic Review. *JAMA Pediatrics, 169*(6), e151025.

Aljazaf, K., Hale, T.W., Ilett, K.F., Hartmann, P.E., Mitoulas, L.R., Kristensen, J.H., & Hackett, L.P. (2003). Pseudoephedrine: effects on milk production in women and estimation of infant exposure via breastmilk. *British Journal of Clinical Pharmacology, 56*(1),18-24.

Aniansson, G., Alm, B., Andersson, B., Håkansson, A., Larsson, P., Nylén, O., Peterson, H., Rignér, P., Svanborg, M., & Sabharwal, H. (1994). A prospective cohort study on breast feeding and otitis media in Swedish infants. *Pediatrics & Infectious Disease Journal, 13,* 183-188.

Arnold, K.C., White, D.E., Caroline, J., & Flint, C.J. (2015). *Association between Raynaud's phenomenon and pregnancy complications.* Retrieved from: www.raynauds.org/wp-content/uploads/2015/05/raynauds-Preg-Study-Results.pdf

Bachrach, V.R., Schwarz, E., & Bachrach, L.R. (2003). Breastfeeding and the risk of hospitalization for respiratory disease in infancy: a meta-analysis. *Archives of Pediatric & Adolescent Medicine, 157*(3), 237-243.

Ball, T.M., & Wright, A.L. (1999). Health care costs of formula-feeding in the first year of life. *Pediatrics, 103,* 870-876.

Ballard, J.L., Auer, C.E., & Khoury, J.C. (2002). Ankyloglossia: assessment, incidence, and effect of frenuloplasty on the breastfeeding dyad. *Pediatrics, 110,* e63.

Balon, A.J. (1997). Management of infantile colic. *American Family Physician, 55(1),* 235-242, 245-246.

Baron, J.A. (1986). Cigarette smoking and prolactin in women, *British Medical Journal, 293,* 482.

Barr, R.G. (1951). Colic and gas. In W.A. Walker, P.R. Durie, & J.R. Hamilton (Eds.). *Pediatric gastrointestinal disease: Pathophysiology, diagnosis and management* (pp. 55-61). Philadelphia: Lippencott.

Belch, J.J., Shaw, B., O'Dowd, A., Saniabadi, A., Leiberman, P., Sturrock, R.D., & Forbes, C.D. (1985) Evening primrose oil (Efamol) in the treatment of Raynaud's phenomenon: A double-blind study. *Throm Haemost, 54*(2),490–494.

Blair, P.S., Heron, J., & Fleming, P.J. (2010). Relationship between bed sharing and breastfeeding: Longitudinal, population-based analysis. *Pediatrics,126*(5), e1119-1126.

Borra, C., Iacovou, M., & Sevilla, A. (2015). New evidence on breastfeeding and postpartum depression: The importance of understanding women's intentions. *Maternal & Child Health Journal, 19*(4), 897-907.

Boyd, C.A., Quigley, M.A., & Brocklehurst, P. (2007). Donor breast milk versus infant formula for preterm infants: Systematic review and meta-analysis. *Archives of Disease in Childhood, 92,* F169-F175.

Cardelli, M.B. (1989). Raynaud's phenomenon and disease. *Medical Clinics of North America, 73(5),*1127-1141.

Chen, M.M., Coakley, F.V., Kaimal, A., & Laros, R.K. Jr. (2008). Guidelines for computed tomography and magnetic resonance imaging use during pregnancy and lactation. *Obstetrics & Gynecology, 112*(2), 333-340.

CMO update 37. (2007). *Soya milk (infant formula).* www.dh.gov.uk/en/Publichealth/Nutrition/Nutritionpregnancyearlyyears/DH_127640

Colson, S., Meek, J., & Hawdon, J. (2008). Optimal positions for the release of primitive neonatal reflexes stimulating breastfeeding, *Early Human Development, 84,* 441-449.

Committee on Toxicity of Chemicals in Food, Consumer Products and the Environment. (2003). *Phytoestrogens and health.* http://cot.food.gov.uk/sites/default/files/cot/cotlsumphytos.pdf

Conrad, P., & Adams, C. (2012). The effect of clinical aromatherapy for anxiety and depression in the high risk postpartum women: A pilot study. *Complementary Therapies in Clinical Practice, 18*(3),164-168.

DeRosa, G. (1981). Prolactin secretion after beer, *Lancet, 2,* 934.

DiGiacomo, R.A. (1989). Fish oil supplementation in patients with Raynaud's Phenomenon: A double blind, controlled, perspective study. *American Journal of Medicine, 86,* 158-164.

Dixon, M., & Khan, L.R. (2011). Treatment of breast infection *British Medical Journal, 342,* 484-489.

Duncan, B., Ey J, Holberg, C.J., Wright, A.L., Martinez, F.D., & Taussig, L.M. (1993). Exclusive breast feeding for at least 4 months protects against otitis media. *Pediatrics, 5,* 867-872.

Dvorak, B., Fituch, C.C., Williams, C.S., Hurst, N.M., & Schanler, R.J. (2003). Increased epidermal growth factor levels in human milk of mothers with extremely premature infants. *Pediatric Research, 54*(1),15-19.

Frost, B.L., Jilling, T., & Caplan, M.S. (2008). The importance of pro-inflammatory signalling in neonatal NEC. *Seminars in Perinatology, 32*(2), 100–106.

Geddes, D.T., Langton, D.B., Gollow, I., Jacobs, L.A., Hartmann, P.E., & Simmer, K. (2008). Frenulotomy for breastfeeding infants with ankyloglossia: Effect on milk removal and sucking mechanism as imaged by ultrasound. *Pediatrics, 122*(1), e188 -e194. Retrieved from: http://pediatrics.aappublications.org/content/122/1/e188.abstract

Goergen, S., & Molan, M. (2009). *The Royal Australian and New Zealand College of Radiologists gadolinium contrast medium (MRI Contrast agents).* Retrieved from: www.insideradiology.com.au/pages/view.php?T_id=38#.VGUqyvmsUtq

Griffiths, D.M. (2004). Do tongue-ties affect breastfeeding? *Journal of Human Lactation, 20*(4), 409–414.

Groer, M.W., & Davis, M.W. (2006). Cytokines, infections, stress, and dysphoric moods in breastfeeders and formula feeders. *Journal of Obstetric, Gynecological & Neonatal Nursing, 35*(5), 599-607.

Grube, MM et al (2015) Does Breastfeeding Help to Reduce the Risk of Childhood Overweight and Obesity? A Propensity Score Analysis of Data from the KiGGS Study. *Plos One.*

Hale, T., & Rowe, H. (2014). *Medications and mothers' milk.* Online access.

Hogan, M., Westcott, C., & Griffiths, M. (2005). Randomised controlled division of tongue tie infants with breastfeeding problems. *Journal of Paediatric & Child Health, 41*(5–6), 246–250.

Hollis, B.W., Wagner, C.L., Howard, C.R., Ebeling, M., Shary, J.R., Smith, P.G., Taylor, S.N., Morella, K., Lawrence, R.A., & Hulsey, T.C. (2015). Maternal versus infant Vitamin D supplementation during lactation: A randomized controlled trial. *Pediatrics, 136*(4), 625-634.

Holmen, L., & Backe, B. (2009). Underdiagnosed cause of nipple pain presented on a camera phone. *British Medical Journal, 339*, b2553.

Howie, P.W., Forsyth, J.S., Ogston, S.A., Clark, A., & Florey, C.D. (1990). Protective effect of breastfeeding against infection. *British Medical Journal, 300*, 11-16, 52.

Inch, S., & Fisher, C. (1995). Mastitis: infection or inflammation? *The Practitioner, 239*, 472-476.

Ip, S., Chung, M., Raman, G., Chew, P., Magula, N., DeVine, D., Trikalinos, T., & Lau, J. (2007). *Breastfeeding and maternal and infant health outcomes n developed countries.* Agency for Healthcare Research and Quality (AHRQ). Evidence Report/Technology Assessment No. 153.

JG Alves, JN Figueiroa, J Meneses, and GV Alves. Breastfeeding Protects Against Type 1 Diabetes Mellitus: A Case-Sibling Study. Breastfeed Med 5 Aug 2011.

Kahl, L.E., Blair, C., Ramsey-Goldman, R., & Steen, V.D. (1990). Pregnancy outcomes in women with primary Raynaud's phenomenon. *Arthritis & Rheumatism, 33*(8),1249-1255.

Kanabar, D., Randhawa, M., & Clayton, P. (2001). Improvement of symptoms in infant colic following reduction of lactose load with lactase. *Journal of Human Nutrition and Dietetics, 14*, 359-363.

KellyMom. (n.d.). *Lactose intolerance.* Retrieved from: http://kellymom.com/health/baby-health/lactose-intolerance/

Kendall-Tackett, K.A., Cong, Z., & Hale, T.W. (2013). Depression, sleep quality, and maternal well-being in postpartum women with a history of sexual assault: A comparison of breastfeeding, mixed-feeding, and formula-feeding mothers. *Breastfeeding Medicine, 8*(1), 16-22.

Kendall-Tackett, K.A., Cong, Z., & Hale, T.W. (2011). The effect of feeding method on sleep duration, maternal well-being, and postpartum depression. *Clinical Lactation, 2*(2), 22-26.

Kernerman, E., & Newman, J. (2015). *Raynaud's Phenomenon.* Retrieved from: www.nbci.ca/index.php?option=com_content&view=article&id=52:vasospasm-and-raynauds-phenomenon&catid=5:information&Itemid=17

Koren, G., Cairns, J., Chitayat, D., Gaedigk, A., & Leeder, S.J. (2006). Pharmacogenetics of morphine poisoning in a breastfed neonate of a codeine-prescribed mother. *Lancet, 368*(9536), 704.

Kramer, M.S., Guo, T., Platt, R.W., Sevkovskaya, Z., Dzikovich, I., Collet, J.P., Shapiro, S., Chalmers, B., Hodnett, E., Vanilovich, I., Mezen, I., Ducruet, T., Shishko, G., & Bogdanovich, N. (2003). Infant growth and health outcomes associated with 3 compared with 6 months of exclusive breastfeeding. *American Journal of Clinical Nutrition, 78*, 291-2959, e837-842.

Kwan ML et al (2004). Breastfeeding and the risk of childhood leukemia: A meta-analysis. Public Health Rep 119: 521-35.

Lactmed database. (2016). Retrieved from: http://toxnet.nlm.nih.gov/cgi-bin/sis/htmlgen?LACTMED

Leppert, J., Myrdal, U., Hedner, T., & Edvinsson, L. (1994). The concentration of magnesium in erythrocytes in female patients with primary Raynaud's phenomenon: Fluctuation with the time of year. *Angiology, 45*, 283–228.

Liu, B., Jorm, L., & Banks, E. (2010). Breastfeeding and the subsequent risk of maternal Type 2 diabetes. *Diabetes Care, 33*(6), 1239-1241.

Lucassen, P.L.B.J., Assendelft, W.J.J., Gubbels, J.W., van Eijk, J.T.M., van Geldrop, W.J., & Knuistingh Neven, A. (1998). Effectiveness of treatments for infantile colic: A systematic review. *British Medical Journal, 316*, 1563-1569.

Ludman, S., Shah, N., & Fox, A.T. (2013). Managing cow's milk allergy in children. *British Medical Journal, 347*, f5424.

Marild, S., Hansson, S., Jodal, U., Odén, A., & Svedberg K. (2004). Protective effect of breastfeeding against urinary tract infection. *Acta Paediatrica, 93*(2), 164-168.

Matthiesen, A.S., Ransjö-Arvidson, A.B., Nissen, E., & Uvnäs-Moberg, K. (2001). Postpartum maternal oxytocin release by new-borns: Effects of infant hand massage and sucking. *Birth, 28*(1), 13-19.

McAndrew, F., Thompson, J., Fellows, L., Large, A., Speed, M., & Renfrew, M.J. (2010). *Infant feeding survey.* Retrieved from: www.hscic.gov.uk/catalogue/PUB08694/Infant-Feeding-Survey-2010-Consolidated-Report.pdf

Metcalf, T.J., Irons, T.G., Sher, L.D., & Young, P.C. (1994). Simethicone in the treatment of infant colic: A randomized, placebo-controlled, multicenter trial. *Pediatrics, 94*, 29–34.

MHRA Codeine. (2015). *Restricted use as analgesic in children and adolescents after European safety review.* Retrieved from: www.gov.uk/drug-safety-update/codeine-restricted-use-as-analgesic-in-children-and-adolescents-after-european-safety-review

Mikiel-Kostyra, K., Mazur, J., & Boltruszko, I. (2002). Effect of early skin-to-skin contact after delivery on duration of breastfeeding: a prospective cohort study. *Acta Paediatrica, 91*(12), 1301-1306.

Mitchell-Box, K., Braun, K.L., Hurwitz, E.L., & Hayes DK. (2013). Breastfeeding attitudes: Association between maternal and male partner attitudes and breastfeeding intent. *Breastfeeding Medicine, 8*(4), 368-344.

Morrell, C.J., Slade, P., Warner, R., Paley, G., Dixon, S., Walters, S.J. et al. (2009). Clinical effectiveness of health visitor training in psychologically informed approaches for depression in postnatal women: Pragmatic cluster randomised trial in primary care. *British Medical Journal, 338*, a3045.

National Institute for Health and Clinical Excellence. (2011). *Food allergy in children and young people: Diagnosis and assessment of food allergy in children and young people in primary care and community settings.* Retrieved from: www.nice.org.uk/guidance/cg116

NHS Introducing Solid Foods. (n.d.). Retrieved from: www.nhs.uk/start4life/solid-foods

NICE Division of Ankyloglossia (tongue-tie) for breastfeeding (IPG 149). (2005). Retrieved from: www.nice.org.uk/guidance/ipg149

Nikodem, V.C., Danziger, G.N., Gulmezoglu, A.M.G., & Justus Hofmeyr, G. (1993). Do cabbage leaves prevent breast engorgement? A randomized, controlled study. *Birth, 20*(2), 61-64.

Owen, C.G., Martin, R.M., Whincup, P.H., Davey Smith, G., & Cook, D.G. 2006). Does breastfeeding influence risk of type 2 diabetes in later life? A quantitative analysis of published evidence. *American Journal of Clinical Nutrition, 84* (5), 1043-1054.

Paton, L.M., Alexander, J.L., Nowson, C.A., Margerison, C., Frame, M.G., Kaymakci, B., & Wark, J.D. (2003). Pregnancy and lactation have no long-term deleterious effect on measures of bone mineral in healthy women: A twin study. *American Journal of Clinical Nutrition, 77,* 707-714.

Paul, I.M., Downs, D.S., Schaefer, E.W., Beiler, J.S., & Weisman, C.S. (2013). Postpartum anxiety and maternal-infant health outcomes. *Pediatrics, 131*(4), e1218-1224.

Pisacane, A., Graziano, L., & Zona, G. (1992). Breastfeeding and urinary tract infection. *Journal of Pediatrics, 120,* 87-89.

Polatti, F., Capuzzo, E., Viazzo, F., Colleoni, R., & Klersy, C. (1999). Bone mineral changes during and after lactation. *Obstetrics & Gynecology, 94,* 52-56.

Porter, R.H. (2004). The biological significance of skin-to-skin contact and maternal odours. *Acta Paediatrica, 93*(12), 1560-1562.

Price, M., & Johnson, M. (2005). Using action research to facilitate skin-to-skin contact. *British Journal of Midwifery, 13*(30), 154-159.

Quigley, M.A., Kelly, Y.J., & Sacker A.S. (2007). Breastfeeding and hospitalization for diarrheal and respiratory infection in the United Kingdom Millennium Cohort Study. *Pediatrics, 119,* e837- e842.

Ramsay, D.T., Mitoulos, L., Kent, J.C., Larsson, M., & Hartmann, P.E. (2005). The use of ultrasound to characterize milk ejection in women using an electric breast pump. *Journal of Human Lactation, 21*(4), 421-428.

Raynaud's and Scleroderma Association. Retrieved from: www.raynauds.org.uk/raynauds/coping-with-raynauds

Rebhan, B., Kohlhuber, M., Schwegler, U., Fromme, H., Abou-Dakn, M., & Koletzko, BV. (2009). Breastfeeding duration and exclusivity associated with infants' health and growth: Data from a prospective cohort study in Bavaria, Germany. *Acta Paediatrica, 98,* 974-980.

Redsell, S., et al. (2015). Systematic review of randomised controlled trials of interventions that aim to reduce the risk, either directly or indirectly, of overweight and obesity in infancy and early childhood. *Maternal & Child Nutrition. 12* (1, 24-38).

Salman, S., Sy, S.K., Ilett, K.F., Page-Sharp, M., & Paech, M.J. (2011). Population pharmacokinetic modeling of tramadol and its o-desmethyl metabolite in plasma and breast milk. *European Journal of Clinical Pharmacology, 67,* 899-908.

Savilahti, E., Launiala, K., & Kuitunen, P. (1983). Congenital lactase deficiency. A clinical study on 16 patients. *Archives of Diseases of Childhood, 58,* 246-252.

Smith, W.O., Hammarsten, J.F., & Eliel, L.P. (1960). The clinical expression of magnesium deficiency. *JAMA, 174,* 77-78.

Thorne, J.C., Nadarajah, T., Moretti, M., & Ito, S. (2014). Methotrexate use in a breastfeeding patient with rheumatoid arthritis. *Journal of Rheumatology, 41*(11), 2322.

Turlapaty, P., & Altura, B.M. (1980). Magnesium deficiency produces spasms of coronary arteries: relationship to etiology of sudden death ischemic heart disease. *Science, 208,* 198–200.

UNICEF UK Baby-Friendly. (2013). *The evidence and rationale for the UNICEF UK Baby Friendly Initiative standards.* Retrieved from: www.unicef.org.uk/BabyFriendly/Resources/General-resources/

Vandenplas, Y., Brueton, M., Dupont, C., Hill, D., Isolauri, E., Koletzko, S., Oranje, A.P., & Staiano, A. (2007). Guidelines for the diagnosis and management of cow's milk protein allergy in infants. *Archives of Diseases of Childhood, 92,* 902-908.

VanderVaart, S., Berger, H., Sistonen, J., Madadi, P., Matok, I., Gijsen, V.M., de Wildt, S.N., Taddio, A., Ross, C.J., Carleton, B.C., Hayden, M.R., & Koren, G. (2011). CYP2D6 polymorphisms and codeine analgesia in postpartum pain management: A pilot study. *Therapeutic Drug Monitor, 33*(4), 425-432.

Wagner, C.L., & Greer, F.R. (2008). Prevention of rickets and Vitamin D deficiency in infants, children, and adolescents. *Pediatrics, 122*(5), 1142-1152.

Webb, J.A., Thomsen, H.S., Morcos, S.K., & Members of Contrast Media Safety Committee of European Society of Urogenital Radiology (ESUR). (2005). The use of iodinated and gadolinium contrast media during pregnancy and lactation. *European Radiology, 15*(6), 1234-1240.

Welborn, J.M. (2012). The experience of expressing and donating breast milk following a perinatal loss. *Journal of Human Lactation, 28*(4), 506-510.

Wessel, M.A., Cobb, J.C., Jackson, E.B., Harris, G.S., & Detwiler, A.C. (1954). Paroxysmal fussing in infancy, sometimes called "colic." *Pediatrics, 14,* 421-434.

Widström, A.M., Lilja, G., Aaltomaa-Michalias, P., Dahllöf, A., Lintula, M., & Nissen, E. (2011). Newborn behaviour to locate the breast when skin-to-skin: A possible method for enabling early self-regulation. *Acta Paediatrica, 100(1),* 79-85.

Wilson, A.C., Forsyth, J.S., Greene, S.A., Irvine, L., Hau, C., & Howie, P.W. (1998). Relation of infant diet to childhood health: Seven year follow up of cohort of children in Dundee infant feeding study. *British Medical Journal, 316(7124),* 21–25.

World Health Organization (WHO). (2000). *Mastitis causes and management.* Retrieved from: www.who.int/maternal_child_adolescent/documents/fch_cah_00_13/en/

Yan et al. (2014). The association between breastfeeding and childhood obesity: a meta-analysis. *BMC Public Health. 14,* 1267.

Zavaleta, N. (2005). Iron and Lactoferrin in milk of anaemic mothers given iron supplements. *Nutrition Research, 15*(5), 681-690.

INDEX

W

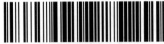

Made in the USA
Charleston, SC
18 January 2017